T0213538

The Pathway to Publishing: A Guide to
Quantitative Writing in the Health Sciences

Stephen Luby • Dorothy L. Southern

The Pathway to Publishing: A Guide to Quantitative Writing in the Health Sciences

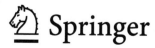

Springer

Stephen Luby
Center for Innovation in Global Health
Stanford University
Stanford, CA, USA
e-mail: sluby@stanford.edu

Dorothy L. Southern
Oxford, England
e-mail: dorothysouthern2016@gmail.com

This book is an open access publication.

ISBN 978-3-030-98177-8   ISBN 978-3-030-98175-4   (eBook)
https://doi.org/10.1007/978-3-030-98175-4

© The Editor(s) (if applicable) and The Author(s) 2022

Open Access   This book is licensed under the terms of the Creative Commons Attribution 4.0 International License (http://creativecommons.org/licenses/by/4.0/), which permits use, sharing, adaptation, distribution and reproduction in any medium or format, as long as you give appropriate credit to the original author(s) and the source, provide a link to the Creative Commons license and indicate if changes were made.

The images or other third party material in this book are included in the book's Creative Commons license, unless indicated otherwise in a credit line to the material. If material is not included in the book's Creative Commons license and your intended use is not permitted by statutory regulation or exceeds the permitted use, you will need to obtain permission directly from the copyright holder.

The use of general descriptive names, registered names, trademarks, service marks, etc. in this publication does not imply, even in the absence of a specific statement, that such names are exempt from the relevant protective laws and regulations and therefore free for general use.

The publisher, the authors and the editors are safe to assume that the advice and information in this book are believed to be true and accurate at the date of publication. Neither the publisher nor the authors or the editors give a warranty, expressed or implied, with respect to the material contained herein or for any errors or omissions that may have been made. The publisher remains neutral with regard to jurisdictional claims in published maps and institutional affiliations.

This Springer imprint is published by the registered company Springer Nature Switzerland AG
The registered company address is: Gewerbestrasse 11, 6330 Cham, Switzerland

Preface

Stephen Luby is a medical epidemiologist who has worked for over 25 years conducting public health research in low-income countries. This effort has included developing the scientific writing skills of early career researchers whom he collaborated with. This guide grew out of his review of dozens of draft manuscripts from novice scientists in Pakistan in the mid-1990s. To avoid writing the same critique into multiple manuscripts, he developed a short list of "most common errors" with explanations of how they should be addressed. This allowed him to refer to manuscript errors more quickly by number, and allowed writers to see a more complete description of the problem than might be typed out when he recognized a familiar error in a new manuscript.

Over the years, these "most common errors" multiplied. While working in Bangladesh, Stephen began collaborating with Dorothy Southern, who edited and organized this rather unwieldy list and integrated explanations and examples from a number of different sources. As Dorothy and Stephen recognized new errors, they incorporated them into the guide. Dorothy also worked to broaden the document to describe the mentor-orientated approach to scientific writing that they promoted in the Centre for Communicable Diseases at the International Centre for Diarrhoeal Disease Research, Bangladesh (icddr,b).

Neither of us is now living in Bangladesh, but we both remain involved teaching scientific writing to early career scientists, especially those working in low- and middle-income countries. We have chosen to publish this as an open access guide so that it can be downloaded at no charge by scientists working in low-resource settings.

The *Pathway to Publishing: A Guide to Quantitative Writing in the Health Sciences* focuses on the unique format and data presentation of quantitative studies in the health sciences. It aims to support and encourage scientists who are actively engaged in quantitative research to write effectively, and so increase the sharing of important scientific results. Since this guide grew out of training public health scientists in Pakistan and Bangladesh, many of the examples are from this context, though the principles apply broadly to clear scientific writing.

Bringing scientific work to publication is a group effort. Scientific writing, like the broader scientific enterprise, is a collaboration based on the exchange of ideas. While this guide is primarily focused on providing support to first authors, it also describes the roles and responsibilities of co-authors. Although the specification of these roles was originally articulated to support the management of scientific writing at icddr,b in Bangladesh, they remain appropriate principles for the Center for Innovation for Global Health at Stanford University and for other collaborative scientific groups.

We hope this guide helps you share more of your useful findings and ideas with international scientific readers.

Stephen Luby
Dorothy L. Southern

Acknowledgments

We are grateful to our many colleagues who provided feedback on prior descriptions of these errors.

We particularly appreciate Laura Kwong's contribution to the section on plagiarism (Error 2.2.2), Robert Fontaine who contributed much of the ideas and examples for Error 7.10 (table layout that impairs comparison), and Robert H. Schmidt who provided the text for the authorship scorecard (Appendix 8).

Contents

Part I
Introduction

Chapter 1
Introduction

1.1 The Pathway to Publishing

Scientific writing is a key skill for researchers. Scientific writing develops critical thinking, helps scientists connect their local results with global understanding, and helps scientists identify appropriate next questions to explore. Increased scientific writing capacity within a research group allows more study results to be shared with the practitioner community and policy makers. More writers mean more work gets published so all members of the scientific team benefit.

However, there are several barriers to publishing: a lack of focus in framing the research question, difficulty in explaining why the study is important (the "so what?" question), inexperience in interpreting data and drawing out its implications, unfamiliarity with the requirements of scientific writing formats, and a lack of clarity and conciseness in the use of English language.

The pathway to publishing, especially when it involves collecting original data, is a long process that begins with the development of a research idea and typically requires years to unfold. Often, a scientific writer's first opportunity as an author will come on a project that was initiated by other scientists. The pathway to publishing process (Fig. 1.1) describes the documents that a researcher might be required to write and the steps along the way to becoming a first author. Sometimes, researchers will address questions of previously collected data or be dispatched by government authorities to conduct an outbreak investigation. In these circumstances, the scientists will not have to work through the long process of securing funding and will begin to work sooner on data analysis and writing.

© The Author(s) 2022
S. Luby, D. L. Southern, *The Pathway to Publishing: A Guide to Quantitative Writing in the Health Sciences*, https://doi.org/10.1007/978-3-030-98175-4_1

Develop research question(s)
Develop a first draft **concept note** outlining the objectives with broadly summarized methods (Appendix 1: Concept note outline)
After co-investigator review, develop a revised concept note including sample size and budget (Appendix 2: Concept note example)
After internal review, develop a **funding proposal**
IF FUNDED
Draft a **study protocol**, based on the funding proposal. (Appendix 3: Critical questions for protocol development)
Secure review from all co-investigators (and from external reviewers if required by the institutional review board)
After responding to all comments and securing co-author approval, submit for institutional review board review
Once approved, implement research activities and collect data
Analyze the data and construct draft tables and figures for the manuscript Share this **framing document** with your senior author (Appendix 4: Framing document) (Appendix 5: Flowchart for review of scientific documents)
Develop a **high-level outline**. Share with co-authors (Appendix 6: High level outline) (Appendix 7: High level outline example)
After responding to all comments, develop the first draft manuscript
Circulate to senior author
Respond to senior author review
When senior author approves, circulate draft to all co-authors
Revise manuscript, responding to all co-author comments
Send revised draft back to co-authors for further review
Revise repeatedly until all co-authors agree the manuscript is ready for journal submission
Submit for institutional clearance
Submit to appropriate journal
Receive peer reviewers' comments and respond appropriately
Re-submit to journal
Congratulations on your first author published manuscript!

Fig. 1.1 The pathway to publishing

1.2 Think-Before-You-Write Approach

To think critically about and start writing any type of scientific paper, use the six-step "think-before-you-write" approach.

1.2.1 Develop a Framing Document

The role of a framing document is to assess if the proposed results and analysis provide a sufficient basis for a useful manuscript. A single study commonly generates multiple manuscripts. A framing document helps to clarify which results belong in which manuscript. A framing document provides early feedback to ensure that the author is on a productive path. Even if there will only be a single manuscript coming out of a study, a framing document helps to clarify the subset of all the data that the study generated that should be included in a manuscript.

The framing document is primarily a communication to be shared among co-authors familiar with the study. It need not include the rationale, a detailed methodological explanation, or any discussion. Think of it as the draft tables and figures for a manuscript with a bit of explanation to clarify framing.

It is however important that the framing document be built upon sound data. So first, double-check the quality of your data and your analysis. If you need help, consult a statistician for input. It is a much better learning experience for the author to conduct the statistical analysis with the coaching of a statistician rather than having the statistician conduct the analysis.

A framing document template is provided in Appendix 4. The framing requires an explicit statement of the objective of the manuscript. A manuscript's objective may be closely aligned or quite different from the objective of the study. The main results should be specified if they either are a simple number or are not readily understood from reviewing the tables and figures.

1.2.2 Focus on the High-Level Outline

After your senior author and other co-authors have confirmed that the analyses included in your framing document would support a manuscript, the next step is to develop a brief high-level outline of the manuscript.

The role of the high-level outline is to sketch out the major components of the manuscript that will support the data analysis included in the framing document. This is an outline that should be no longer than 1500 words (excluding the tables, figures, and references). Full sentences are not necessary. A format is provided in Appendix 6.

Keeping the document short helps the author focus on the key elements of the manuscript. It provides opportunity for early input on the scope and framing of the key ideas. Because a short document takes less time for authors to produce and less time for co-authors to review, it generates prompt feedback on key ideas and so supports a faster path to publication. Using this approach prevents authors investing weeks or months developing full draft manuscripts that are off target with pages and pages of prose that need to be discarded.

High-level outline benefits	
For writers	For reviewers
Bullet points focus on thinking skills rather than writing skills	Content is easy to see and to understand
Provides framework to guide the thinking process	Short, concise format
Allows continuous input and revision	Critical results stand out
Saves many hours developing manuscript sections that will not be included	Easy to change the framing if necessary

1.2.3   Use the "Most Common Errors"

Use the "most common errors" listed in *A Guide to Quantitative Writing in the Health Sciences* as a method for reviewing and editing the first and all subsequent drafts of a scientific paper. All the errors listed in the guide have been repeatedly identified in draft scientific papers written by early career writers. These errors range from problems with punctuation, referencing, and data presentation to not understanding the difference between association and causality. Examples of the "most common errors" are provided along with alternative or better options. Reviewing a paper using the "most common errors" has several benefits for both the writer and the reviewer.

The "most common errors" benefits	
For writers	For reviewers
Eight categories of errors	Covers most errors
Provides more detailed explanations than a reviewer could provide on every point	Quick, easy system
	Saves time. No need to repeat explanations
Real illustrative examples	Puts the responsibility on the writer to find the
Systematic learning process	corresponding link to the error and to read and learn about it

1.2.4   Understand Authorship and Mentoring Responsibilities

Scientific writing is a collaborative effort. The framing document and high-level outline provide an initial opportunity to identify the first author and co-authors. Inclusion on an author line indicates one's contribution to scientific work. Authorship is an important professional credential. The norms for the ordering of authors varies by discipline. In economics, authors are listed alphabetically. In the life sciences, the position of first author, second author, and last author carries specific responsibilities outlined below.

First Author
- Conducts the analysis but may receive substantive input/support from statistical colleagues on complex elements of the analysis
- Constructs the framing document with tables and figures and shares with senior author
- After revision and approval from senior author, shares the framing document with tables and figures with co-authors
- Drafts a <1500-word, high-level outline
- After revision and approval from senior author, seeks input from co-authors
- Develops multiple high-level outline drafts by responding to all reviewers' comments
- Drafts the manuscript
- Follows all the instructions for a draft manuscript as noted in Error 2.5 (not using standard draft manuscript form)
- After revision and approval from senior author, seeks input from co-authors
- Develops multiple drafts of manuscript by responding thoroughly and thoughtfully to co-authors' feedback (avoids Error 8.2)
- If a co-author is a government official, the first author:
  - Asks the co-author about the process for securing government approval for manuscript submission
  - Provides the necessary documents to request approval

- Once senior author and co-authors agree, submits the manuscript to a journal
- Circulates submitted draft
- Keeps co-authors informed of all progress on the submission
- Circulates response from editors and comments from reviewers to all co-authors
- Drafts response to reviewers' comments
- Circulates response to reviewers' comments along with a marked-up version of the manuscript (to highlight changes) to all co-authors for feedback

Senior Author
- Usually, the senior author is a topic expert who has published first authored work related to the topic of the paper. Leveraging this knowledge and expertise, the senior author ensures that the paper is framed to make a meaningful contribution to the scientific literature.
- The senior author is listed last on the manuscript and often serves as the corresponding author.
- When the first author is an early career scientist, the senior author assumes the role of primary reviewer and assists the first author in:
  - Drafting the author line
  - Selecting an appropriate journal

- Deciding who should be the corresponding author
- Identifying external reviewers for journal submission (though first author should generate candidates; see Error 8.9)
- Performs the reviews of the initial drafts of the framing document with tables and figures
- Decides when the framing document with tables and figures is sufficiently developed that it would benefit from review by all co-authors
- Performs the reviews of the initial drafts of the high-level outline
- Decides when the high-level outline is sufficiently developed that it would benefit from review by all co-authors
- Reviews the initial drafts of the draft manuscript
- Decides when the draft manuscript is sufficiently developed that it would benefit from review by all co-authors
- Decides when the draft manuscript is ready for submission to a journal
- Assists the first author in finalizing the author line. For example, if a proposed co-author was included in the initial draft but never provided any input to the draft manuscript and so does not meet the international criteria for authorship, this co-author would generally be dropped from the author line
- Carefully reviews the first author's responses to external reviewers' critiques
- Decides when the revised manuscript and responses to external reviewers' critiques are sufficient and the manuscript is ready for resubmission

Second Author
- The second author is generally the person who made the next largest contribution to the manuscript after the first and senior author although this designation is sometimes used to denote particularly important institutional collaborators.
- The particular role of the second author should be discussed with the senior author. The second author may have additional responsibilities in addition to standard co-author roles including:

  - Drafting sections of the manuscript
  - Performing the role of primary reviewer
  - Functioning as senior author
  - Functioning as the corresponding author

Co-author
- Provides thorough, substantive review of the high-level outline
- Provides thorough, substantive review of the draft manuscript
- Drafts specific sections of the manuscript in one's particular area of expertise and contribution as requested by the first or senior author
- Ensures that the elements of the study that are within their area of responsibility and expertise are accurately and appropriately reflected in the manuscript
- Ensures that framing of scientific arguments and references to the literature that are within their area of expertise are sound and appropriate
- Assesses if they meet the criteria of co-authorship

- Assesses if they are sufficiently comfortable with (1) the quality of the work, (2) the integrity of study implementation and analysis, and (3) the conclusions that it reaches that they are willing to accept public responsibility for its content
- Co-authors can opt out of inclusion on the authorship line during any of the drafts, but they should do so before submission to a journal. It is unprofessional to remove one's name after submission because it signals to the journal editor that you were not consulted prior to submission

Getting feedback from the senior author, second author, and co-authors is crucial to ensure that a scientific paper clearly describes a valid methodology and communicates convincing results.

In the best-case scenario, all co-authors discuss and agree on the responsibilities and contributions early on, preferably during the development of the protocol when the roles of the investigators are specified. Practically, however, which specific findings will ultimately support a manuscript and so how many manuscripts will be written and how each should be framed are usually impossible to anticipate before the data are analyzed. In addition, the composition of the scientific team and interest and availability of potential authors is often different by the time the data are available compared with the original plan, and so authorship typically needs to be revisited.

Once the data are available, the project principal investigator reviews the earlier planning around authorship and leads a discussion with co-investigators that revisits the earlier conversation and works to reach decisions about framing and assignment of first author responsibilities. Usually, there is no shortage of first author writing opportunities. Principal investigators are commonly eager to identify co-investigators willing to lead a manuscript. Often, project co-investigators will suggest a manuscript that they are particularly interested in leading.

Gift Authorship   Assigning someone authorship or designating someone a first or a senior author when they have not completed these roles is dishonest. Sometimes, a skilled author views granting another person first authorship when they have not discharged the responsibilities of first authorship an appropriate gift for other contributions to the project. This may seem like a generous expression of gratitude, but it is a rather patronizing hollow token. It is a much more valuable gift for seasoned authors to invest the time to develop less experienced writers and to work closely with them so that they can accomplish the first author responsibilities and have legitimately earned the role. This process generates skills that allow the new author to advance their scientific writing career, a genuinely useful gift.

Authorship Conflicts   Conflicts over whom to include as an author and their position on the author line are common. Sometimes, a person who was influential in securing funding or in providing institutional permission to participate in the study insists on inclusion in the author line and/or insists on being named a senior or first author (Error 8.3). One way to reduce these conflicts is to include language in institutional agreements and in the protocol that international standards of authorship will be used to determine authorship contribution. The International Committee of Medical Journal Editors provide clear guidelines for authorship (www.icmje. org) (Error 8.3). It is helpful to enter conversations with an author line framed using standards for assigning authorship aligned with the International Council of Medical Journal Editors or other authoritative source. The authorship scorecard (Appendix 8) provides a useful quantitative tool to develop and defend an author list.

1.2.5   Structure the Writing and Feedback Process

Constructive criticism and focused comments from co-authors are crucial to help a first author refine and improve their work. Your initial and subsequent drafts should be reviewed first by the senior author or primary reviewer and then by your other co-authors (Appendix 5).

First authors should share each of the documents they have drafted: the framing document, the high-level outline, or a draft manuscript. They should expect multiple reviews and revisions but in a culture of trust and openness. Reviewers should provide timely feedback. They may deploy the "most common errors" to highlight areas in need of further work.

A review and feedback schedule should be agreed on to ensure the pathway to publishing can be covered in the shortest time possible. Long delays in giving comments and suggestions to improve a scientific paper can de-motivate the writer and delay the dissemination of meaningful research. A suggested time frame for review is as follows:

Structured feedback timeline	
Type of document	Reviewed within
Concept note	5 working days
Protocol	5 working days
Framing document	5 working days
Conference abstract	3 working days
Poster	5 working days
High-level outline	10 working days
Draft manuscript	10 working days
Reponses to journal editors and reviewers	5 working days

The first author also has a responsibility to continue to dedicate time regularly to the manuscript. Writing well enough so that editors and reviewers agree that your work is a novel and useful contribution to the global scientific literature requires substantial ongoing time commitment from the first author. The biggest difference between people who are authors and people who aspire to be authors but do not achieve this aspiration is that authors dedicate substantial time to writing. A long delay in developing the next draft of a paper means the article loses its developmental momentum and potentially even its relevance to the global scientific discussion.

Co-authors usually have multiple ongoing projects and will move their attention to other papers. Although a strict schedule for producing revised drafts is difficult to prescribe because substantive critiques may require a deep and critical review of the literature, more in-depth statistical analysis, or additional laboratory work or data collection, writers should commit substantial time each week to revising and improving their drafts.

1.2.6 Responding to Co-author Comments

Remember, it normally takes 10 working days to get all the reviewers' comments on a draft manuscript. Indeed, it is a good practice when circulating a draft manuscript to request input by a specific date. Ten working days is a reasonable timeline. If you provide less time than this, you risk communicating a lack of respect for the time of your co-authors. Similarly, when you are a co-author, it is a responsibility to provide input within a reasonable time frame so that the development of the manuscript is not delayed.

Read all reviewers' comments carefully before starting to revise to get an overall picture of how others interpreted your paper. Oftentimes, it is useful to read the comments all through once to get a general idea of the criticism (and feel the pain that not every reader loved every decision you made). Then after a day or two, go back through each of the comments carefully. Often, there are a number of major changes you will want to make to your manuscript. We recommend implementing those changes in a revised manuscript. After you have implemented the major changes, you can then proceed with line by line to comments and suggestions.

When preparing for a line-by-line revision, it is useful to consider the comments from all of the reviewers. This may be complicated because some reviewers will provide comments on the version you circulated, ignoring comments made by others. Oftentimes, reviewers will provide comments on a version that others have already commented on. Sometimes, this creates divergent drafts with different reviewers responding to a version of the manuscript with a different set of previous reviewers.

The Compare feature of Microsoft Word can combine various drafts so that all of the comments are together on each page. This can be helpful, but sometimes, this squeezes so many comments on a page that you can only see the first line of the comment. One tip to make these readable is to insert page breaks at frequent intervals so that for each section of the manuscript that you are reviewing, all of the reviewer comments are readable.

Combining drafts will not always work well because the Compare feature requires that you accept one set of revisions before adding other drafts. This conflates your original text with reviewers' revisions. In addition, if some reviewers provide handwritten comments on a printed or scanned version, there is no direct way to assemble these into a single document. In these cases, you can take the various versions of the commented manuscript and either print each one out or display them on multiple computer screens. The goal is to be able to easily read every reviewer comment on a sentence or paragraph before making a decision on how to revise it.

Of course, not all comments or suggestions will be useful or even correct. You, as first author, need to make the decision about which comments and suggestions to accept and how to revise. If there is a major comment that you do not agree with, you should explain why either by inserting a comment (using track changes) or by stating the reason in the accompanying email or in an attached document. If you have a lot of reviewers and a lot of comments, you can draft a document on "Co-author suggestions I did not take." You can organize this document by the co-author. Describe their comment and the reason you did not make the suggested change. This allows the co-author to jump immediately to your response to their critique and so efficiently decide whether more conversation would be fruitful.

1.2.7   Summary of the Think-Before-You-Write Process

A first-authored scientific publication develops your scientific reasoning, bolsters your credentials as a scientist, shares your organization's work, and contributes to global scientific knowledge.

Following this six-step "think-before-you-write" approach helps all authors work efficiently to generate high-quality manuscripts. Spending initial time developing and collecting feedback from a framing document and a high-level outline saves countless hours in the long run. Responding to the "most common errors" identified by reviewers quickly improves the quality of the drafts. Sharing the draft versions of your paper with co-authors on a timely basis ensures you make steady progress toward publication.

1.3   The Writing and Publishing Process

1.3.1   Converting Preliminary Work into a Manuscript

Oftentimes, authors have presented the core findings of their planned manuscript in another format perhaps as a verbal or poster presentation, as a report for a funding agency or government authority, or as a thesis for an academic degree. These efforts can be quite helpful in developing a manuscript. They often advance analysis and framing and provide a forum for the author to collect feedback on their work. With all the effort to develop a report or thesis, it may seem that just a few hours work will be required to reformat the work into a manuscript. However, more commonly, even with this preliminary work, developing a manuscript is a substantial task.

A thesis or a report has a different audience than a journal article. This different audience calls for a somewhat different focus, a different level of detail and meticulous attention to previously published work and careful scientific reasoning. A funder is likely to be primarily interested in how the study addressed the project objectives. A thesis may require a particular format and attention to specific issues depending upon the department or institution issuing a degree. By contrast, a scientific manuscript should be framed around the novel information that you are presenting to the international scientific community and how this new knowledge connects with prior ideas and findings previously published in the scientific literature.

Instead of beginning with your draft report, we recommend beginning to draft a manuscript for a scientific journal by drafting a framing document (described above in Sect. 1.2.2). This allows both you and your senior author to step back and consider what are the primary new data that this work will present to an international scientific audience. Once the framing document is approved, then draft a high-level outline and circulate this first to your senior author and then to co-authors. A few rounds of iterative development, especially of the outline for the discussion and introduction, can help clarify how the narrative of your study will be framed for an international scientific audience. Once co-authors have approved the content of the high-level outline, proceed to develop a full-draft manuscript. For the draft manuscript, you will be able to copy and paste from a prior report or thesis, but this will build out an outline that is now custom designed for a scientific journal article.

1.3.2 The Peer Review Process

Peer review is a distinguishing feature of scientific publication. Prior to publication, any scientific manuscript presenting original data must be reviewed by peer scientists, who have the opportunity to raise questions and criticism. Only after an editor is satisfied that concerns of these peers have been addressed is a paper published. Although the process of peer review is imperfect, international scientific discourse is improved by this systematic process. It reduces publication of work with profound flaws in methods or scientific reasoning. It results in better articles being available for other scientists to read.

Editor's Decision When you submit your manuscript to a journal, an editor assesses whether the article fits within the scope of the journal, would be of interest to readers, and avoids obvious methodological errors. If the editor is satisfied that the article meets these and potentially other conditions, then the editor sends the article for external peer review. Reviewers are selected based on their subject matter expertise, which is generally judged by their published work. Reviewers cannot have any association with the proposed work. Authors commonly suggest potential reviewers (see Error 8.9).

Reviewers provide feedback to the editor on the strengths and weaknesses of the submitted manuscript. They recommend to the editor whether or not the work should be published. The quality of these reviews is variable. Some excellent reviews provide thoughtful detailed comments. Addressing these reviews improve the manuscript. These external reviews can function like a good co-author review but often with the benefit of some distance from the project and deep engagement with related literature. Other reviews are vague and not particularly useful. A third group are hostile and unprofessional. These can take various forms, but the criticism is not constructive. They might misconstrue the paper and obsess over tangential issues.

The editor considers the reviews and usually makes one of several decisions. The editor may accept the manuscript asking only for minor changes to address some of the issues raised by the reviewers. The editor may be inclined to accept the paper if the authors can address substantive concerns. The editor may be undecided but willing to consider a revised draft that addresses the concerns raised by the reviewers. Finally, the editor may be persuaded by the reviewers that there are fundamental problems with the paper or with its appropriateness for the journal and choose to reject it.

Author's Decision Once the editor makes a decision, the authors face a decision. If the editor remains interested, first consider the issues raised by the reviewers. If major revisions are required and you believe they would improve the paper, begin by addressing these concerns. These major issues may require additional analysis, new figures or tables, or substantial revisions to framing.

Once you have addressed the major revisions, then began to work through each comment raised by each reviewer. Develop a clear, thorough response document. This document should stand on its own so that the editor can read it from beginning to end without needing to refer back to the manuscript to understand what the issues are and what changes were made. Unless it was only a minor grammatical change or typographical error, text that was revised should be included as quotations in the response document (avoid Error 8.2.1). Regardless of the tone of the reviewer, the tone of the response document should be professional. Even in a highly critical review, look for areas to agree with the reviewer even if only on a minor point, and note when you have made the suggested change. On areas of substantive disagreement with the reviewer, make a thorough and carefully reasoned case for your approach and your interpretation. You are aiming to persuade the editor that your approach and interpretation is sound.

Early career scientists should send a draft of their response to review document with a clean and a marked-up version of their revised manuscript to their senior author for review. Often, there will be a few drafts back and forth between the first and senior author before the senior author is satisfied that the response to review is well enough developed that it would be appropriate to ask co-authors to provide their perspective. All co-authors are publicly accountable for the work, so it is important that they all have the opportunity to review the substantive concerns raised by the reviewers and the proposed revisions. It is best to resubmit the revised manuscript by the deadline specified by the editor. Because these responses require a few rounds of feedback with the co-author team, it is important to begin working on these responses shortly after receiving the external reviews. If you are unable to meet the deadline for resubmission requested by the editor, ask for an extension with a specific deadline that you can meet.

If the editor rejects the manuscript, do not become disheartened. Rejections are common in the pathway to publishing. If the manuscript was sent for external review, these reviews can provide helpful perspective on how a few other readers view your work. Addressing reviewer input often improves the manuscript. Occasionally, external reviewers will identify a previously unrecognized fundamental problem with the manuscript. If so, you can choose to abandon the effort to bring the manuscript to publication. More commonly, a manuscript rejection simply reflects a judgment by an editor that this work is not of sufficient interest to the journal's audience, and so your task as an author is to continue to work with your manuscript and identify a more appropriate home for it.

Perhaps the most important issue to face after rejection of the manuscript is where you will submit it next (see Error 8.5). With authors using computer-based searches to identify relevant work, a solid paper will be identified and cited repeatedly even if it is published in a journal that does not have a particularly high-impact factor. Solid journals that provide high-quality reviews are excellent ways to bring your work to publication and advance your career.

If you believe the editor has made a substantial error in judgment, perhaps because they have accepted a harsh reviewer's critique that is easily answered, you can ask for the decision to be reconsidered. Most journals have a formal process to reconsider rejected manuscripts. Occasionally, this is successful, but it risks delaying eventual publication. Time spent appealing to an editor who has already rejected the article is time that could be spent submitting the manuscript to a new journal.

Preprints Preprints of unpublished manuscripts that have not yet been peer-reviewed are increasingly common in the natural sciences though they have long been used in economics. Preprint repositories commonly used in the health sciences include arXiv, bioRxiv, and others. Advantages of posting your submitted manuscript on a preprint server include that it makes these draft results available to other groups. If there is a particular urgency in getting your findings out, this can make these results available months before a peer-reviewed publication. The availability of a draft manuscript on a preprint server allows you to point to your submitted work as part of a grant application. It communicates to the proposal reviewers that your work is well advanced. Indeed, if they are interested, they can even pull the submitted manuscript and read it. Posting your work to a preprint server also allows you to assert priority on the publication of a novel finding.

Disadvantages of posting your draft manuscripts to a preprint server include that these manuscripts are not peer-reviewed and so do not have the same credibility as peer-reviewed publications. They are not indexed as consistently in bibliographic search databases that scientists routinely use to identify relevant work. They are a less credible citation than published work. Some high-impact journals will not consider manuscripts if the details have previously been made publicly available. These journals are interested in actively participating in the dissemination of work they publish through broader journalistic channels. If you are submitting to a high-impact journal, check their policy prior to making your submitted version widely available.

1.4   The Scientific Writing Style

Use the six "S's" below to guide your scientific writing:

Structured
Write under the guidance of the high-level outline, knowing where the logic starts from and where it is going.

Sequential
A key characteristic of good scientific writing is reader centricity. Take the reader by the hand through the sequence of thoughts, step-by-step, without any leaps or missing links in the development of the ideas. Give the reader information when they need it in a logical sequence that anticipates their questions. This facilitates their ability to interpret and critique the information.

Simple
Use simple words to explain what is meant. Imagine trying to explain the concept to a layperson. Don't use technical or statistical jargon. If you find you about to write or type a word you wouldn't use in everyday conversation, stop and simplify.

Short
Use short sentences containing only one idea in each. Split complex sentences. Cut unnecessary information elements and only include those data that relate to the point of your paper. Do not include data just because you collected them. If it is an interesting result but is not directly related to the focus of the paper, it should not be included in the paper. Remember, "if it's only nice to know, it ought to go." If it is a clarifying point supported by a lot of data analysis, consider including it as supplementary information.

Strong
Use the verb as the center of gravity of your sentence. If the verb is weak, the sentence is weak. For example, instead of "we did an interview," write "we interviewed." Use active voice instead of passive. For example, instead of "the study was conducted," write "we conducted the study." With active voice, the subject does the action of the verb, which implies more immediacy and transparency (see Error 5.3).

Specific

Say clearly and exactly what you want to say. Don't use qualifiers, which are imprecise and judgmental (Error 6.3). Avoid words such as "very," "rather," or "much." Choose adjectives carefully. Don't use adjectives that imply subjectivity and/or emotion (Error 5.5), for example, "It *was a very large outbreak." What does very mean?* How big is <u>large</u>? Science readers prefer numbers.

Open Access   This chapter is licensed under the terms of the Creative Commons Attribution 4.0 International License (http://creativecommons.org/licenses/by/4.0/), which permits use, sharing, adaptation, distribution and reproduction in any medium or format, as long as you give appropriate credit to the original author(s) and the source, provide a link to the Creative Commons license and indicate if changes were made.

The images or other third party material in this chapter are included in the chapter's Creative Commons license, unless indicated otherwise in a credit line to the material. If material is not included in the chapter's Creative Commons license and your intended use is not permitted by statutory regulation or exceeds the permitted use, you will need to obtain permission directly from the copyright holder.

Part II
Most Common Errors

Chapter 2
General Research and Writing Practices

2.1 Insufficient Knowledge of the Literature

The first step in developing a scientific document is not writing but thinking and reading. Good authors are good readers. To write a good paper, you need to develop your own critical thinking, creative thinking, and understanding. You need to have read and critically considered what others have previously reported.

This error can take several forms, such as not having read the relevant literature, not understanding and integrating the work of others into the paper, or ignoring work that threatens or contradicts your findings or beliefs. Authors need to understand what has been previously published on the topic in order to frame the research question and to highlight novel elements of their contribution. If the author lacks sufficient interest in the topic to read about it in detail, then the author is not well positioned to convince readers to be interested in that topic. Failure to demonstrate familiarity with the literature and understanding of the topic also jeopardizes an author's credibility.

Remember, experts in the field will be reviewing your paper. Your initial drafts will be reviewed first by your primary reviewer and then by your co-investigators, co-authors, and research group head. When you submit a manuscript to a journal, it will be peer-reviewed. If you don't find the most up-to-date relevant information, then a reviewer is likely to do it for you, resulting in embarrassment and/or rejection of your paper.

An author needs to understand and communicate what the state of knowledge in the field is and describe what your paper adds to what is already known. You are trying to advance the field of knowledge, not just duplicate it. You cannot do this unless you are intimately familiar with what is already known. This should transcend, "There is almost no data on this subject in Bangladesh," the implication being that anything I say will be an improvement. While prior work may be limited, you need to look at similar settings or even dissimilar settings and see what other

© The Author(s) 2022
S. Luby, D. L. Southern, *The Pathway to Publishing: A Guide to Quantitative Writing in the Health Sciences*, https://doi.org/10.1007/978-3-030-98175-4_2

researchers have found. What are the principal ideas, explanations, and data that are relevant to your particular paper?

If you cannot answer the question, "What does this paper add to what is already known about this subject in the literature?," then you are not ready to write the paper. Expect to spend many days finding relevant articles and reading them critically before you can understand and then communicate clearly what new information or idea your paper adds. Different electronic search engines can help you identify different articles: By default Google Scholar lists the number of times an article is cited and so can help you identify articles that are influential, while PubMed can be set to list the most recent articles first.

When conducting a literature review, it is, at times, acceptable to put together a concept note or a first draft of a protocol by reviewing abstracts of journal articles. However, to cite information in a paper for submission to a journal, we recommend reading the manuscript for two reasons. First, a scientific argument that is sufficiently refined to be included in a peer-reviewed scientific article requires a nuanced understanding of the work you cite, a level of specificity that is unavailable from an abstract. Second, there may be data or an argument in a cited article that directly challenges a central idea you are presenting in your paper. If you fail to note it and address the implications for your paper, you risk losing credibility in the minds of readers and reviewers.

Finally, the excuse of "I couldn't get the paper" is not acceptable in the arena of international scholarship. It is more difficult when articles are behind pay walls, but with persistence, nearly any article can be secured. Online resources and collaboration with other institutions and even directly writing authors can secure helpful sources.

Examples of the error		Alternative, better options	
X	Key studies in the field are not quoted.	✓	Search the literature carefully.
X	The studies quoted do not represent the best or the latest studies.	✓	Update literature search, and identify "citation classics".
X	Study findings are misrepresented.	✓	Read all cited papers fully, not only the abstracts.

2.2 Insufficient Citations

Citations in the text that point to a list of references at the end of your article provides a standardized approach to acknowledge the sources of information and ideas that you have used. It allows readers to locate and review the basis of your arguments.

Learn and use a reference management software. Options include EndNote, Mendeley, Zotero, Papers, JabRef, and many others. Reference software helps you track the source of the information and ideas that contribute to your own scientific understanding.

Keep track of your sources in a physical or electronic logbook during your research. When you identify useful ideas or information, include a citation and reference in your notes.

2.2.1 Not Providing a Reference to Support an Observation

Scientific arguments require specificity. All statements that are not common knowledge or do not flow directly from your data require a citation within the text that points to a reference that supports the assertion. This requirement flows from the central importance of empirical findings in constructing and defending scientific arguments. Regular citation also reinforces the social construction of scientific understanding.

For novice scientific authors, this requirement may seem odd or stilted. We don't use this in our normal conversation. Even journalists commonly make general assertions without citations and references. Peer-reviewed scientific literature is different.

Consider the statement *"It is estimated that by 2050, half of all deaths will be a result of environmental mismanagement."* Who made such an estimate? What is the basis of this estimate? Is this one person's opinion (Error 2.3.3)? If this estimate was based on a model, what are the model assumptions? Such general statements may be common in popular discourse, but in scientific writing, the reader needs to know the basis of each of your assertions. Readers can then judge whether this assertion and so the scientific argument within your manuscript is credible or not.

Examples of the error		Alternative, better options	
X	Pneumonia is a major public health problem in India.	✓	In 2018, pneumonia was the leading cause of death among children in India (ref).
X	Handwashing is effective against diarrheal diseases.	✓	Community level interventions that promoted handwashing have been associated with reduced incidence of childhood diarrhea (ref).

2.2.2 Plagiarism

Plagiarism is presenting other people's work as your own. This is a particularly serious error. It has destroyed the reputation and careers of many scientists. Web search tools make it increasingly easy to detect plagiarism.

A particularly egregious form of plagiarism is copying text word for word from another source and not attributing the source. Anytime an author quotes >3 words from a source, you should use quotation marks as well as a citation. More commonly in scientific writing, authors paraphrase the ideas and results from other articles and add a citation.

Authors can commit plagiarism unintentionally when they are pulling ideas together for a scientific manuscript or proposal. Authors might copy text from various articles and paste this text into a working document to help assemble relevant observations and ideas. Authors may subsequently insert this text into a draft manuscript losing track that the specific words originated from someone else. To avoid this error, whenever you copy text from another article, use quotation marks when you paste it into your own notes, and include a citation that points to the original author's work.

Example of the Error
Built environment has direct and indirect effects on mental health* and *poor quality housing increases psychological distress* and *insufficient daylight is associated with increased depressive symptoms* (Evans 2003).
Cited reference:
Evans, G. W. The built environment and mental health *J Urban Health* 2003 Dec;80(4):536–55.
Abstract of Cited Reference
The built environment has direct and indirect effects on mental health. High-rise housing is inimical to the psychological well-being of women with young children. *Poor-quality housing* appears to *increase psychological distress*, but methodological issues make it difficult to draw clear conclusions. Mental health of psychiatric patients has been linked to design elements that affect their ability to regulate social interaction (e.g., furniture configuration, privacy). Alzheimer's patients adjust better to small-scale, homier facilities that also have lower levels of stimulation. They are also better adjusted in buildings that accommodate physical wandering. Residential crowding (number of people per room) and loud exterior noise sources (e.g., airports) elevate psychological distress but do not produce serious mental illness. Malodorous air pollutants heighten negative affect, and some toxins (e.g., lead, solvents) cause behavioral disturbances (e.g., self-regulatory ability, aggression). *Insufficient daylight is* reliably *associated with increased depressive symptoms*.
*The ***bold italic*** format reflects direct quotations from the published work.
Ⅹ This is an error because the author is directly quoting from a source but using neither quotation marks nor a citation.

Alternative, Better Options
As Evans notes, "the built environment has direct and indirect effects on mental health . . . (and) poor quality housing appears to increase psychological distress. . . and insufficient daylight is associated with increased depressive symptoms" (Evans 2003).
Poor quality housing that provides little daylight worsens psychological health (Evans 2003)

Science is a social enterprise. Scientific writing requires that we give credit to others who have informed our ideas. A less egregious form of plagiarism than unattributed direct quotation involves using the ideas of others but failing to cite the source of these ideas and so presenting the ideas as your own. Because scientific discourse builds on the ideas and findings of others, scientific authors aim to situate their work within broader scientific discussion. It is important to cite the sources that led to the specific framing of the issues presented in your work.

Some journals are concerned with "self-plagiarism." There are two related concerns here. First, most scientific manuscripts are framed as presentations of original data. Duplicate publication of the same work in more than one journal typically violates both the norms of science and the rules of individual journals. Journals want to ensure that original work is genuinely novel. When publishing multiple articles from the same underlying study, sometimes some analysis, for example, the baseline comparison of characteristics between intervention groups, may be of interest to readers of multiple papers. If you are presenting some results that have been previously published, it is important to make this clear within the manuscript.

A second concern is that authors often sign over copyright to journals. Thus, if they are using the same language they have used before, they are actually using copyrighted material of a copyright they may no longer own. At its extreme, a concern with avoiding self-plagiarism means that an author would need to rewrite the methods section using different words even when producing the tenth paper describing various outcomes of a randomized controlled trial. This can become absurd. Best practice is to refer to a prior article that provided details and then offer a succinct summary.

(Thanks to Laura Kwong for her assistance in drafting this section on plagiarism.)

2.3 Weak Citations

Scientific reasoning is based upon what can be observed in the world. Authors support scientific arguments by pointing to various observations. An original scientific paper includes new observations and argues that they inform broader understanding. Although it is sometimes appropriate to cite specific arguments, ideas, or theoretical models, the most common citations are observations reported by other scientists. Three common forms of the weak citation error are:

2.3.1 Citing a Secondary Source

In this form of the error, the author cites an article that cites the original observation. Standard scientific practice is to cite the primary observation. It is a flagrant error if you cite an article that makes a similar point to the argument you want to make in your article, and the article that you are citing perhaps, in its introduction, cites the primary articles. Avoid this error by simply citing the primary article.

Sometimes, it is appropriate to cite meta-analyses or other reviews, but the best practice in most cases is to cite the relevant primary literature even if it requires multiple citations. Citing the primary literature points directly to the empirical basis of the assertion. It specifies where critical readers should look if they are interested in further exploring these data. It also signals to the reader, who may know the literature very well, that you are also familiar with the relevant literature. If you are citing work that people are not so familiar with, but it is important to your argument, this can be an important pathway to support a somewhat different interpretation than the dominant interpretation. This process encourages creative connections, critical thinking, and productive scientific argumentation.

2.3.2   Presenting Conclusions Rather Than Data
from References

Scientific understanding advances by reasoned interpretation of observation. Indeed, an essential difference between scientific discourse and nonscientific discourse is this reliance on observation as the cornerstone of argument. Thus, if you want to make a persuasive scientific argument, you need to present the core data, not just a person's conclusion from that data.

Example: *A baseline evaluation of the quality of sexually transmitted disease case management was conducted in five areas of Chennai, in 2012, and it was found that there is an urgent need for health-care providers to adopt the syndromic approach to STD treatment.*

In this example, the cited study may well have concluded that the health-care providers' performance was so poor in detecting and treating sexually transmitted diseases that a move to a syndromic approach was the best option. But if this is being presented as evidence that sexually transmitted disease diagnosis and treatment were poor, why should a scientific thinker have to accept the judgment or opinion reached by someone else? Accepting another's judgment without personally evaluating the data upon which that judgment is based is nonscientific reasoning. Nonscientific reasoning is out of place in a scientific manuscript.

Consider the alternative, better option: *In a baseline evaluation of the quality of sexually transmitted disease case management conducted in five areas of Chennai in 2012, 74% of persons presenting with symptoms of sexually transmitted diseases were given treatment that differed from World Health Organization guidelines.*

Now, the reader is no longer being asked to accept the interpretation of the author of the original study or of the author of the present manuscript. The reader has been given the primary observation that forms the basic unit of reasoning and so can either accept it as appropriate to the idea being developed or not. With the data, the reader can follow the author's reasoning.

2.3.3   Arguing from Authority

An argument from authority asserts that readers should accept a statement as true because of the authority of the person who spoke it. In everyday life, we depend upon arguments from authority to help navigate the world. We believe the auto mechanic who tells us our car will not start because the battery is too weak to hold a charge. We believe the attorney we consult who suggests that adding a specific clause in a contract will prevent subsequent legal problems. Arguments from authority are commonly used in many religious traditions and among journalists.

A distinctive feature of scientific reasoning, by contrast, is that it eschews arguments from authority and instead asserts that statements are credible because of the empirical evidence that supports them. Scientists do not believe statements because they were uttered by a prestigious university or government official. Scientific reasoning requires evidence.

Examples of the error		Alternative, better options	
X	Many experts emphasize that shared toilets are the only solution for urban slum residence.	✓	Because of severe constraints on space, shared toilets will continue to be a common option in urban slums the foreseeable future.
X	Daniel Kahneman, a Nobel prize winning economist, notes that human decision-making is frequently illogical.	✓	Numerous formal assessments find that human decision-making is frequently illogical (references).

2.4 References Not in Standard Style

There are many times that a scientist is required to exercise creativity and ingenuity. Writing endnotes is not one of those times. Endnotes for manuscripts have standard formats well detailed in the "Uniform Requirements for Manuscripts submitted to Biomedical Journals" (www.icmje.org).

Various reference management software programs are available that assist in tracking and reporting references including EndNote, Zotero, Mendeley, Papers, JabRef, and many others. They allow an author to quickly insert bibliographical information. They automate renumbering references when text is resequenced after copying and pasting. They can quickly convert from one reference format to another if a journal requires a different reference format.

2.4.1 Varying Citation Format

Different journals use different formats for citations and references. There are two general approaches. Most journals sequentially enumerate the references in the order that they appear in the narrative. Different journals that use sequential numbering require that the citations within the text be displayed differently. Some prescribe that numbers be displayed within square back brackets. Others want numbers in parentheses. Others request superscripts. Some journals want reference numbers to precede periods or commas. Others want them to follow.

The other general approach is to list references at the end of the article alphabetically based on the first author's last name. The in-text citations include one or more of the authors' name and the year of publication.

When drafting a manuscript, look up your target journal's reference format and use it. If you are writing a proposal or other piece of work that does not have a set format, then use a format that is easy for readers to understand. If you are space constrained, choose an enumerated format.

Do not mix formats that is sometimes using author's last names in parentheses and other times using numbers. Sometimes, copying and pasting from different documents create this problem. It risks confusing readers and making it difficult for them to connect to your references.

2.4.2 Not Proofreading References Prior to Submission

None of these reference management programs work flawlessly. All have their strengths, weaknesses, and idiosyncrasies. Prior to submission, the first author needs to carefully review each reference, ensure that it is complete, that capitalization is appropriate, and that there are no spelling or other obvious errors. When circulating a submission-ready manuscript to co-authors for their sign off, the references should be proofread. Submitting sloppy references communicates a lack of attention to detail. Journal editors prefer to engage authors who attend to details.

If response to further review requires any changes in the references, this often requires redeploying the reference management software that will likely replicate many of the earlier errors. These can be minimized by making corrections to the source references within the management software, but because of imperfections in reference management software, this is insufficient. Prior to resubmission, the references need to be proofread again.

2.5   Not Using Standard Draft Manuscript Form

Most journals have specific instructions for manuscripts submitted to them, usually detailed in their website under "Instructions to Authors." However, as a good starting point, the following generic style would be appropriate for a first draft manuscript sent to co-authors for review.

1. Format a title page to include:
   - The title of the article
   - First name, middle initial, and last name of each author (check the journal to see if they have a limit on the number of authors)
   - Each author's institutional affiliation as a superscripted note
   - Targeted journal(s)
   - Main text total word count
   - Abstract total word count
   - Key words

2. Include an abstract in the format and within the word length of the targeted journal. If the journal choice is uncertain, then include a structured abstract (text separated into sections labeled background, methods, results, and conclusion) of no more than 250 words.

3. The main text of the article should be in the traditional format of introduction, methods, results, and discussion (IMRAD). Different disciplines and different journals have different norms regarding the appropriate length of an article. The main text should not exceed the word limit for your target journal. Shorter articles are particularly attractive to most journal editors. If the journal does not suggest a limit, look at the length of articles that they generally publish. A manuscript that is too long risks discouraging reviewers, editors, and readers. By contrast, if a paper is too short, editors and reviewer can request that more information be included.

4. The manuscript should be double-spaced using a common font size 12. This provides more space for comments for reviewers of both the paper and electronic version.

5. The narrative text should be in a single column. Don't try to make it look like a formatted two-columned journal article. It makes it harder to review electronically, and it is also not the form it needs to be in for a specific journal submission.

6. Indent the first word of each paragraph one tab width (0.25–0.5 inch), or skip a line between paragraphs to signal the reader that this is the start of a new set of ideas.

7. Align text to the left. (Avoid Error 4.8.)

8. Insert the acknowledgments after the discussion. Then add references up to the limit permitted by the journal.

9. Tables and/or figures should be placed after the references. Journals often limit the number of tables and/or figures.

2.6 Repeating Information

Editors of scientific manuscripts prefer succinct writing. Don't repeat ideas. Say it well and say it once. A useful strategy to reduce repetition is by carefully considering the logic of your arguments in presenting the ideas so that they build progressively. If a point is so important that you want to ensure that reader see it, then include it in both the body of the paper, and the abstract, which is a summary of the manuscript.

A subtle version of this error is including both proportions of a dichotomous outcome in a results table (see last example).

One situation where a modicum of repetition may be appropriate is in the development of some ideas in the discussion when it is appropriate to link the development of these ideas to specific study results and/or to issues of study rationale raised in the introduction.

However, in a linked discussion, the important point is not to repeat the words but rather to make a logical connection between what was raised earlier and the discussion about to take place. Thus, a short recall, without quantitative details, is sufficient. Some journals, including *The Lancet*, want the first paragraph of the discussion to summarize the main results.

Examples of the error		Alternative, better option
X	"Disease X causes XXX deaths annually worldwide" used in the first paragraph of the introduction and in the first paragraph of the discussion.	Don't repeat an idea. Say it well and say it once. If you are unsure about where to mention it, review Error 3.2 that clarifies the respective roles of each section of a
X	Full repetition of results, with quantified data and statistical tests in the discussion section.	manuscript to identify the most suitable place.
X	Household pays for electricity Yes 3 (10%) No/don't know (90%)	Household pays for electricity 3 (10%).

2.7 Labeling a Scientific Document as "Final"

Avoid the word "final" in the title or the description of any scientific document. Scientific thinking is always open to revision. To call a document final implies either dogmatic close-mindedness or naiveté, both characteristics that are inconsistent with a genuine scientific outlook.

Examples of the error		Alternative, better options
X	Attached is the final version of the protocol.	Attached is the version of the protocol approved by the Institutional Review Board.
X	Here is the final version of the manuscript.	Here is the published version of the manuscript. (Who knows, there may be letters to the editor or subsequent insight that requires further revisions?).

2.8 Characterizing an Observation as "The First"

Scientists take pride in identifying novel observations. Galileo was the first person to see moons around Jupiter. Darwin was the first to both notice the very high variation of bird species on tropical islands and to suggest that this variability was best explained by evolution of species. Watson and Crick were the first to identify the structure of deoxyribonucleic acid (DNA). Part of that task of writing a manuscript is to explain to the readers what is new about the information that is being presented and how this new information changes or refines global scientific understanding. In this context, many authors will assert that their scientific findings are "the first." However, there are three problems with describing one's scientific findings as "the first."

1. These assertions can create controversy and ill feeling with some scientists writing venomous letters to the editor disputing the claim of primacy. Such ill feelings do not help scientific understanding progress. Indeed, if one of your subsequent papers or research funding proposals is then reviewed by one of these

scientists who felt slighted by not being appropriately recognized in your earlier work, you risk receiving an unnecessarily devastating review that does not fairly consider the merits or your work. Indeed, many journal editors (e.g., those at the Lancet) will not publish claims of first primarily because they prefer to avoid such nonproductive ego-driven controversy.

2. Every observation can be described as a first if there are sufficient qualifications. Thus, the assertion of "first" is not, in itself, meaningful, for example, "This is the first time that hepatitis E virus has been confirmed using advanced molecular methods in environmental water supplies in Shakira District during the dry season at night using locally trained staff." Asserting that something is "first" does not communicate why it matters.

3. These assertions distract from useful explanations of how these observations contribute to global scientific understanding. If a health condition has been found in the other 10 countries where it has been looked for, then saying that this is the first time this has been recognized in Bangladesh tells us more about the interest of Bangladeshi scientists in this condition and the funding available to work in this area than about the health condition itself or the situation in Bangladesh. It does not tell readers why this observation is important.

Like all rules in the guide, this one is not absolute. An occasional claim of first may be defensible and help to clarify to the reader how to interpret the results, but >95% of scientific articles are best written without any claim to "first."

Examples of the error		Alternative, better options	
X	This is the first time that an association between hepatitis C infection and carcinoma of the liver has been demonstrated in Liberia.	✓	The link noted between hepatitis C and liver carcinoma in this population in Liberia provides further evidence of the importance of hepatitis C as a leading cause of hepatocellular carcinoma globally. It suggests that for a low-income country like Liberia, preventing the transmission of hepatitis C may be the most cost-effective way to prevent liver carcinoma.
X	This is the first time that Nipah virus antibodies have been identified in dogs in Bangladesh.	✓	Nipah virus infects a wide range of mammals. Earlier studies in Malaysia identified dogs with evidence of Nipah virus infection, but similar to our findings in Bangladesh, dogs appear to be dead-end hosts rather than the reservoir of the infection.

2.9 Errors in Reasoning

Scientific reasoning is central to interpreting our scientific results and to sound, persuasive communication with our colleagues. There are many ways that scientific reasoning can go awry. Indeed, one of the main benefits we derive from co-authors and external reviewers critically reviewing our manuscripts is that they criticize our reasoning and so help us to improve it. Some criticisms of scientific reasoning reflect different interpretations of reported observations in the published scientific literature. What follows, however, are more formal errors in the structure of argument.

2.9.1 Casual Assertion of Causality

Scientists take the idea of causality very seriously. Indeed, much scientific work is centered around developing causal hypotheses that explain a relationship between characteristics and exposures in the world and subsequent outcome. When a scientist concludes that a particular chemical exposure caused illness, this is an argument that is based on careful observation, a biologically plausible mechanism, systematically collected data that demonstrates a statistical association, and rejection of alternative explanations including bias and chance [1].

By contrast, when nonscientists speak they tend to be much less careful in their assertion of causality. Business journalists commonly assert that the stock market went down because, for example, the weather was cold, a large company reported disappointing quarterly results, or investors were concerned about recent political developments. Similarly, politicians will assert, for example, that the reason crime has increased is because there are too few police officers. Sport journalists and fans will assert that the reason the home team lost the soccer match is because they did not take their opponents seriously. Each of these assertions may or may not reflect a genuine causal relationship, but none of the people making the assertion is offering a rigorous scientifically persuasive argument.

Such casual assertions of causality, which might be acceptable in casual conversation political speech or daily journalism, is not acceptable in scientific writing. Thus, especially in the introduction and discussion sections of the manuscript, it is critical for your credibility as a scientist not to assert causality unless there is rigorous evidence to support this assertion.

Examples of the error		Alternative, better options	
X	Banning overnight poultry storage at live bird markets have been found to reduce influenza H9N2 circulation substantially in Hong Kong.	✓	After overnight poultry storage at live bird markets in Hong Kong was banned, influenza H9N2 circulation decreased among market poultry.
X	Due to higher temperature, the number of non-cholera diarrhea cases also increased among the individuals with lower educational attainment, non-concrete roofs, and unsanitary toilets.	✓	As temperatures increased, the number of non-cholera diarrhea cases also increased among individuals with less education, non-concrete roofs and unsanitary toilets.

Examples of the error		Alternative, better options	
X	Development project implementation also faltered, the reasons being financial constraints that produced cost overruns and procurement delays, foolhardy recruitment of under-skilled personnel and ill-planned career management, and imprecise delineation of the respective roles of development planning and supporting agencies.	✓	Fewer than 10% of development projects achieved their target objectives. Commentators suggest that the factors that most likely contributed to this underperformance included financial constraints that produced cost overruns and procurement delays, recruitment of under-skilled personnel and ill-planned career management, and imprecise delineation of the roles of development planning and supporting agencies.

2.9.2 Assuming Association Is Causality

Much scientific work aims to identify associations between different phenomena. For example, is a particular exposure (drinking raw date palm sap) associated with a particular outcome (developing Nipah virus infection)? When we construct 2×2 tables or evaluate if there are different mean values between different groups, we are exploring whether there are associations within our data. An important element of our data analysis is to identify relevant associations within our data.

However, just because we find an association, this does not mean that the exposure caused the outcome. For example, if our analysis shows that people who have a lower income have a higher incidence of tuberculosis compared to people who have a higher income, it would be an error in scientific inference to conclude that low income causes tuberculosis infection. Consider for a moment what mechanism we would be asserting. Does the individual *Mycobacterium* have receptors that only attach to the alveolar cells of persons who have an income less than $100 per month? Does the individual *Mycobacterium* wait to see how much money someone spends a month before deciding whether or not to infect him? In this example, low income is better considered an indicator of an environment that puts certain people at risk rather than a cause. For example, people who have low income more commonly have poor nutrition, and this poor nutrition reduces the capacity of the body to defend itself from an infection from *Mycobacterium*. Additionally, people with low income tend to live in more crowded settings where it is easier for respiratory diseases to spread from one person to another. Thus, there is an association between wealth and tuberculosis, but the causal mechanism is a deeper underlying mechanism.

There are a number of other reasons that we might find associations between exposures and outcomes in our data. Three common reasons for associations in our data are bias, chance, and confounding. There are entire books written on each of these topics, and we encourage you to read them. However, when it comes to interpreting your data, any time you see an association, you should be asking yourself the following: What is underlying this association? Is there bias? Could this have arisen by chance? Is this a marker of confounding?

Scientific writing is most persuasive when it invokes a thoughtful, conservative interpretation of association. When discussing an association in the result section, for example, one should never use language that asserts the relationship is causal. In the results, you are only presenting the data and identifying associations.

The argument that an association is causal is an argument that should consider the potential mechanism of action; the possibility that the association is a result of bias, chance, or confounding; and results from other studies including different types of evidence that supports a causal mechanism. An assertion of a causal relationship is an argument that should be made in the discussion section; indeed, such an argument is often the major point of the discussion section.

2.9.3 Assuming Reported Behavior Reflects Actual Behavior

Research in the health sciences often considers human behavior, what people do, and what might influence what they do. Scientific study of human behavior requires deciding how to assess behavior. Usually, the easiest and least expensive approach is simply to ask study respondents how they behave. This can be appropriate and useful, but considerable literature illustrates that compared with actual practice, people generally overreport socially desirable behavior and underreport stigmatized behavior. Scientists should not take reported behavior at face value but consider the likelihood that the reported behavior is not accurately reflecting actual behavior [2]. These considerations are an important aspect of how we interpret our results and so should be considered in the discussion and the limitations.

Sometimes, we use research methods that permit us to directly observe behavior. Although the presence of an observer has been repeatedly demonstrated to alter behavior, observed behavior is often less biased compared with reported behavior. Nevertheless, even scientists who study observed behavior must keep in mind the difference between behavior when an observer is present and the behavior that occurs when people are not being observed.

For example, scientific studies comparing reported handwashing behavior to observed handwashing behavior consistently demonstrate that reported handwashing vastly exceeds observed handwashing [3–5]. Indeed, the differences are so great that reported handwashing behavior is not a valid proxy measure of handwashing practice. Similarly, the handwashing literature provides strong evidence that the presence of an observer markedly increases handwashing [6–9].

In scientific narrative when referring to behavior that has been studied by other researchers or when describing your own work, it is important to keep in mind the deep biases associated with reported behavior. Therefore, when describing behavior, it is useful to clarify whether the behavior was observed or reported.

Examples of the error		Alternative, better options	
X	After the intervention, respondents were less likely to defecate in the open.	✓	After the intervention, fewer respondents reported defecating in the open.
X	In Bangladesh, the rate of exclusive breastfeeding in the first 6 months is 64%.	✓	In the 2011 Bangladesh Demographic and Health Survey, 64% of mothers reported exclusively breastfeeding their children during the child's first 6 months.

2.9.4 Confusing Imperfect Recall with Recall Bias

Human memory is imperfect. If you ask a colleague what they ate for lunch 17 days ago, most would be unable to provide an accurate response. We do not remember all of our experiences. This is imperfect recall. Imperfect recall does not necessarily constitute a bias. Recall bias occurs when different groups of people within the study are likely to remember experiences differently. For example, assume you are conducting a case-control study exploring risk factors for leg fractures. If the injury occurred 2 weeks previously, and you ask people what they were doing in the minutes preceding the injury, cases, that is, people who had experienced a fracture, are much more likely to have carefully considered the events that led up to the fracture and so are likely to recall details of what type of shoes they were wearing, where they were, and what the visibility and footing was. By contrast, if you ask controls about their precise exposures at the same time of day 2 weeks previously, they are much less likely to recall rich details of their experience. Thus, there may be systematic differences in the recall of cases and controls, not because their exposures were different but because their recall of events is different. This is recall bias. All study subjects have imperfect recall. If there is no reason to believe that this recall will differentially affect reports of exposures or outcomes, it should not be labeled as recall bias.

Examples of the error		Alternative, better options	
X	Since the data on exposures to sick poultry was collected by interview, there is a risk of recall bias.	✓	Although our study subjects likely did not recall all of their exposures to sick poultry, because people in this community do not consider sick poultry to be a risk factor for human illness, we would not expect any bias.

2.9.5 Confusing Absence of Recognition with Absence

Authors should not blithely assume that all occurrences of a phenomenon of interest are known to science and reported in the scientific literature. Many events of scientific interest are neither recognized nor recorded in the scientific literature.

Examples of the error		Alternative, better options	
✗	Mortality in ducks and geese as a result of highly pathogenic avian influenza H5N1 infection had never occurred in Bangladesh.	✓	Mortality in ducks and geese as a result of highly pathogenic avian influenza H5N1 infection had never been confirmed in Bangladesh.
✗	The last of the four Nipah outbreaks from India was in 2019.	✓	The last recognized outbreak of Nipah in India was confirmed in 2019.

2.9.6   Asserting Seasonality with a Single Year of Data

Asserting that a phenomenon that occurs at different frequencies in different seasons of a single year is due to seasonality is an error in scientific inference. This is an error because it assumes a pattern when no repetitive pattern has been observed. With only a single year of data from South Asia, for example, only one rainy season was observed. Cases may have increased during the rainy season because a new strain of the pathogen was introduced into the community, a strain that the community did not have immunity against. The strain may have been introduced during the year of observation during the rainy season, but the following year, a new strain might be introduced at a different time of year. We are much less prone to scientific error and have much more credibility if we draw conclusions conservatively from our data. Multiple years of data that show a similar pattern provide a stronger case to assert that the variability in the observation over time is associated with seasonal patterns.

So what should we do if we have 1 year of data and see more cases in the rainy season than in the dry season? It is reasonable in the discussion section to note that the cases were more common in the rainy season, but multiple years of data would need to be observed to see if this is a seasonal pattern.

2.9.7   Drawing Conclusions Using Confirmation Bias

Confirmation bias refers to the human tendency to see patterns in the world that are consistent with previously held beliefs [10]. It is a particularly pernicious bias for scientists because we strive to bring forward new information and to draw sound conclusions.

Confirmation bias often affects scientists when we look at our data and see the patterns that we expect. For example, if people in the intervention group reported less illness, then the data makes sense to us, and we don't dig deeper. By contrast, when we find an association that is unexpected, for example, that disease is more common among people who received the intervention, then we carefully reevaluate the evidence. We check to see if we made a coding error in the analysis or if there was some way the question was framed that might have confused respondents. In short, we invoke a double standard of accepting results that confirm our preconceptions and working to identify problems with evidence that runs counter to our expectations.

Another common manifestation of confirmation bias in science is interpretation of borderline *p*-values. If the point estimate of an association is in the direction that supports the unifying theory that the author is proposing, but the *p*-value is 0.10, authors commonly assert that "borderline result that supports this interpretation." By contrast, if the association is not consistent with the author's favored interpretation, the association is more likely to be left out of the manuscript, ignored in the narrative results, or dismissed as "not significant."

Confirmation bias is so deeply rooted in our human capacity to see patterns in information and the incentives that scientists have to find interesting associations that it is difficult to avoid. A benefit of peer review is that reviewers may not share the authors' preconceptions and so offer alternative interpretations of the data.

As an author, consider the risk of confirmation bias in your interpretation. Seriously consider the strengths and weaknesses of alternative interpretations. Consider the limitations in your data and available data in supporting the most likely interpretation. A conclusion that is based on evidence while also conceding weaknesses and alternative interpretations is more persuasive to a scientific audience.

Examples of the error	Alternative, better options
X — The evidence supports that pesticides contributed to the elevated lead levels among mother.	✓ — The evidence that pesticides contaminated with lead were associated with elevated blood levels is mixed. We found a strong association with reported use of a particular brand of pesticide and blood lead levels, but when we later collected samples of this pesticide, those samples did not contain lead. It is possible that lead arsenate intermittently contaminates commercial pesticides, but further study will be needed to assess this.
X — We found no association between child nutritional status and risk of infection.	✓ — Both well-nourished and poorly nourished children were at risk of infection. Indeed, we found no association between child anthropometric measures and risk of infection though the number of observations were small so we had limited power for this assessment.

2.10 Constructing a Multivariate Model Using Only Statistical Criteria

Scientists are commonly interested in understanding how multiple factors interact to produce a particular outcome. Much of our research efforts are aimed at clarifying these causal pathways. When scientists explore statistical associations between exposures and outcome, they are usually striving to understand if there is an underlying causal connection.

Real-world causal pathways of health outcomes are characteristically complex. Multiple factors generally need to be present (e.g., there is a pathogen in the environment, there is a person who is exposed to the environment, the person is susceptible to the infection). In addition, causal pathways typically have sequences where one exposure must precede another in order for the effect to occur. For example, the pathogen must be present in the environment before the person enters the environment. We are much more likely to add insight to global scientific understanding of underlying causal pathways if we seriously reflect on the likely underlying causal mechanism and then construct our investigations and our data analyses to query these pathways.

All too commonly, analysts simply dump all their exposure variables into a multivariate model and use backward elimination to identify those exposures that are most strongly associated with the outcome and then offer this as a final model. This approach provides no consideration for the potential that two variables may be measuring the same underlying characteristic. It also invokes an implicit causal structure that all the exposures occur simultaneously and without interacting with each other to generate the outcome. This is a naïve and unlikely map of the way processes unfold in the world [11].

A better approach is to develop a causal model that explicates how the scientist believes the various factors are likely to co-produce the outcome and then use this conceptualization to decide which factors to test in the model. There is considerable scholarship on directed acyclic graphs that provide graphical support to help illustrate proposed causal paths and the impact of confounding and temporal sequencing [12, 13] The researcher's proposed causal model can be included as a figure in the paper. This way, readers can follow the hypothesized causal map and understand the judgments used in building a multivariate model.

This is a very different approach than large machine learning efforts that aim not to detect causal relationships but rather to find associations and then use those associations to predict subsequent activity. This type of prediction algorithm has been remarkably successful at identifying patterns in marketing data. In some settings, this widespread search for association in large data sets have been used to identify unexpected associations that may be worth further exploration. This approach remains uncommon among scientists who generally strive to elicit causal understanding. The statistical approach employed should align with the analyst's aspiration.

Examples of the error		Alternative, better options	
X	Tobacco use and male sex are highly correlated (1/34 female respondents reported regular tobacco use as compared to 11/16 males); therefore, although both characteristics meet the specified criteria for inclusion in the final model, only male sex is included.	✓	Tobacco use and male sex are highly correlated (1/34 female respondents reported regular tobacco use as compared to 11/16 males); because tobacco use is known to affect taste (the primary outcome), it was included in the model and sex was dropped.
X	We used univariate logistic regression to select predictor variables significant at the $p < 0.2$ level for inclusion in the full model. We used sequential backward elimination of variables with the weakest association to reach the final model of variables all with $p < 0.05$.	✓	Exposures were grouped in four blocks following the conceptual model: (1) attitude, (2) knowledge, (3) school facilities and programs, and (4) practices. We performed bivariate analysis between exposures and outcome to calculate crude association. We further considered only those exposures associated with outcomes with a $p < 0.2$. We then conducted multivariable analysis among the exposures within each block including confounders identified in the conceptual model. We retained exposure within each block associated with an outcome at the $p < 0.05$ level. We then built an overall multivariate model by using exposure variables from each block that were associated with school absence at the $p < 0.05$ level and which captured most of the measurement.

Open Access This chapter is licensed under the terms of the Creative Commons Attribution 4.0 International License (http://creativecommons.org/licenses/by/4.0/), which permits use, sharing, adaptation, distribution and reproduction in any medium or format, as long as you give appropriate credit to the original author(s) and the source, provide a link to the Creative Commons license and indicate if changes were made.

The images or other third party material in this chapter are included in the chapter's Creative Commons license, unless indicated otherwise in a credit line to the material. If material is not included in the chapter's Creative Commons license and your intended use is not permitted by statutory regulation or exceeds the permitted use, you will need to obtain permission directly from the copyright holder.

Chapter 3
Content of Quantitative Papers

3.1 Improper Focus or Format of Title and Abstract

For your article to become a part of global scientific discussion, people need to read it. Your article's title should be devised so that it interests potential readers to look more closely at the abstract and the article. The title should communicate the topic that the article engages and the approach the authors used to investigate it. It should be descriptive and specific. Some journals require that the type of study, for example, "randomized controlled trial" or "observational study," be included in the title.

Less commonly, some journals encourage titles that also communicate the primary finding. Some authors, especially in economics and qualitative reports, include clever phrases that capture a central notion of the paper.

Check the specific "Instructions to Authors" for your target journal, and note the permissible length of the abstract and whether they require a structured abstract that uses subheadings or an unstructured abstract without subheadings. As most readers will only read the abstract, it is important to craft your abstract so that it communicates the essential information within the word limit.

The abstract must stand alone. It must tell the reader why the topic is important, what the researchers did, what they found out (the most important results and data from the study), and how these findings contribute to knowledge. Do not cite references or use abbreviations. In an unstructured abstract, methods and results can be merged if this improves the narrative flow.

To develop a structured abstract, follow the sequence in Appendix 9

- Background: Explains the rationale for conducting the study, that is, why is this study question important? The last sentence in the background should state the objective of the abstract/manuscript. If space limitations are severe, and there is only sufficient space for a single sentence of background, the one sentence should be a statement of the objective.

© The Author(s) 2022
S. Luby, D. L. Southern, *The Pathway to Publishing: A Guide to Quantitative Writing in the Health Sciences*, https://doi.org/10.1007/978-3-030-98175-4_3

- Methods: Summarizes how the study was carried out. Describe the study population, and explain the key techniques used to generate the primary results reported in the article. For each result, check that you have included a corresponding method.
- Results: Presents the main findings of the study as specific quantitative results. Include raw data with percentages, measures of association, and either confidence intervals or p-values.
- Conclusion: Explains what these results mean, that is, what their broader implications are for science or for public health. They may support specific public health action or specific next steps in research. This is <u>not</u> a summary. Do not repeat results.

3.2 Confusing the Role of Introduction, Methods, Results, and Discussion

The standard structure that most journals prefer for a quantitative scientific paper typically includes the introduction, methods, results, and discussion (IMRAD). The IMRAD structure is explicitly recommended in the "Uniform Requirements for Manuscripts submitted to Biomedical Journals" (www.icmje.org). The content of each of these sections is ruled by conventions that help readers quickly understand the article. The introduction explains why the research question addressed in the manuscript is important, the methods describe how the study was conducted, the results present the findings, and the discussion interprets the results.

These conventions allow the reader to quickly look for the information they are interested in if they choose to read selectively (a common practice). See Appendix 6 for more clarification about what to include in each section.

Examples of the error		Alternative, better options	
✗	Distracting details in the introduction section	✓	Avoid lengthy background on the general topic. Direct reader toward the research question or problem statement.
✗	Replicating the level of detail of the study protocol in the methods section of the manuscript	✓	Focus on key considerations that allow the reader to understand what was done. Do not spell out methods that generated results that are not presented in the manuscript. Add an appendix if there are technical details that a specialist interested in replicating the work would want to know.
✗	Too many details in the results section	✓	Narrow down on a set of results that are key for the conclusion. Supplementary tables and figures can be included in an appendix.
✗	Rambling unstructured discussion	✓	Follow the outline for a discussion (Appendix 6). Identify and succinctly defend your primary claims and their connection to the published scientific literature.

3.3   Not Writing the Methods Section in Chronological Order

The methods section typically involves explaining a number of interrelated activities. A common error is a description that jump back and forth among various components. This risks confusing the reader.

The first part of the methods section for a public health paper is commonly a brief description of the study site and population to explain the context. Then the method section explains in detail the study activities that were performed in sequential chronological order (Appendix 1). Chronological order is standard in narrative and so easy for readers to understand. Departing from chronological order risks confusion.

In a protocol, the methods are written in future tense as these are planned activities. In a manuscript, the methods section is always in past tense to tell the reader what the researchers did.

Example of the error	Alternative, better option
✗ Field research workers will make a monthly promotional visit to all intervention households to educate the primary caregivers about benefits of drinking safe water and to promote the proper utilization of intervention products. We will randomly select 1800 households in five regions, 360 in each. In each follow-up visit, the team also collected stored water from all households who received NaDCC tablets and tested for residual chlorine by using a digital colorimeter. We will provide a 10-liter storage container and 33 mg chlorine (NaDCC) tablets in 600 households, only a 10-liter container in 600 households, and the remaining 600 households will receive no intervention.	✓ Put research and data collection activities into chronological order, and use past tense. • We randomly selected 1800 households in five regions, 360 in each. • We provided a 10-liter storage container and 33 mg chlorine (NaDCC) tablets in 600 households, only a 10-liter container in 600 households, and the remaining 600 households received no intervention. • Field research workers made a monthly promotional visit to all intervention households to educate the primary caregivers of the child about benefit of drinking safe water and to promote the proper utilization of intervention products. • In each follow-up visit, the team also collected stored water from all households who received NaDCC tablets and tested for residual chlorine by using a digital colorimeter.

3.4 Not Emphasizing Steps Taken to Protect Human Subjects

When describing how ethical considerations were addressed by the study team, a writer can misplace the emphasis by first citing that it was approved by a specific human subjects review committee. This sequencing mistakenly implies that the cornerstone of ethical practice is approval by a review committee.

Instead, lead off this section by describing key activities undertaken by the study team to conduct an ethical study. Only the last sentence, somewhat as an afterthought, should confirm that all of these procedures, which the study team developed and carefully and systematically implemented, were reviewed and approved by an appropriate committee. The idea is that the study team acted as moral agents; they neither delegated the ethical conduct of the study to an external group nor simply sought the permission of some institutional authority.

Example of the error		Alternative, better option	
✗	Our study protocol was approved by the ethical review committee of Aga Khan University. Before collecting data, we obtained written informed consent from each adult study participant in the household.	✓	We obtained written informed consent from the adult study participants in each household. The study protocol was reviewed and approved by the ethical review committee of Aga Khan University.

3.5 Listing Interpretations, But Not Defending One in the Discussion

The role of the discussion section is to explain what the results mean. Sometimes, it is tempting to list all the possible interpretations and "let the reader choose" which is the most reasonable. This is an abrogation of the responsibility of the author. As the person who analyzed the data and knows the study, you are in the best situation to explain what the most likely interpretation is and defend it.

It can be useful to mention other important potential interpretations, but the authors should clearly state what they believe the data means and why. For example, the reader who looks at the following text has no idea which of these interpretations is the most plausible.

Example of the error		Alternative, better option	
✗	The difference between the commuting rate and the injury rate may be because men are more likely than women to exhibit risky behavior, particularly not waiting for the bus to stop, hanging on side and climbing on the roof, and running to catch the bus. It could also be explained by a different gender mix on buses during the observation period in these high-risk areas than at other times, or perhaps there are fewer males injured by buses, but this is more than compensated by a disproportionate number of males injured from motorcycles.	✓	Our study found a higher injury rate among men than women. Although we cannot rule out bias in our observations, we did find, consistent with other research on risk taking (ref, ref, ref), that males were more likely to exhibit risky behavior, particularly not waiting for the bus to stop, hanging on side and climbing on the roof, and running to catch the bus.

3.6   Not Fully Explaining Limitations

The objective of a section on limitations is not to list all aspects of the study that could be improved with infinite money and flawless data collection tools in a perfect world. Instead, this section identifies limitations in the inferences that can be drawn from the study. There are four rules for discussing study limitations:

1. State only the most serious limitations. Don't list every possible problem. Although a thesis advisor may be interested in them, a journal reader is not.
2. Focus solely on limitations to scientific inference. It is not the role of a limitation section to list all the shortcomings in the study, all of the issues that you would manage differently given another opportunity in a perfect world. It is not a place to talk about your limitations as an investigator, the limitations of the funding agency, or the limitations of the institutional environment where the study was conducted. Rather, the limitation section should be strictly focused on the limitations to scientific inference that can be drawn from the study.
3. Explain the limitation. Don't just label it. Instead of writing "one of our limitations is selection bias," discuss how you enrolled subjects and how this may result in an unrepresentative study estimate.
4. Discuss how you interpret the data in the light of this potential problem, for example, "it is unlikely that this procedure substantially affected our results because…."

Example of the error		Alternative, better option	
✗	Our study was limited by focusing on only one subdistrict, and so the results might not be generalizable.	✓	Our study focused on only a single subdistrict and so is not representative of the whole country, but the level of economic development, the percentage of the population engaged in agriculture, and the seasonal availability of water is fairly typical of the country.

Example of the error		Alternative, better option	
✗	We did not have sufficient funding to test all of the specimens.	✓	We found no differences between children and adults, but this evaluation was based on a small enough subset of specimens that we had limited power to evaluate modest differences.
✗	Our study was limited by its small sample size	✓	The association of illness with date palm sap consumption was unlikely to be due to chance, but because the outbreak only affected 12 people, we had limited statistical power to identify other potentially important exposures with smaller effect sizes.

3.7 Writing Generic Recommendations

Only make recommendations that your data can support. They should be applicable to the specific context. For example, avoid suggesting interventions in low-income countries that require a level of national income and government capacity equivalent to that of Western Europe (Error 3.11.1).

Generally, recommendations should not simply call for "more research." Such generic calls appear self-serving and do not guide the field. By contrast, it is very useful to reflect on what was learned through your study and identify for the global scientific community (including funding agencies) the one or two important research questions that should next be addressed. Don't provide a laundry list of everything you think should be done. Usually, you should make no more than two practical recommendations.

Recommendations have to be carried out by someone or some agency. Useful recommendations give clear statements about who the actor is, what they should do, and when. Within public health and other applied sciences, scientists are often asked to actively assist in translating scientific knowledge to practical advice for nonresearchers. A mechanism to achieve this is through knowledge translation briefs or one-page summaries of key messages and evidence-based recommendations for action derived from the research results. Aimed at the right institutions and interest groups, evidence-based information and recommendations can inform national policy and programs to address important problems.

3.8 Presenting New Data in the Discussion

The role of the discussion is to tell the reader what the authors believe the results mean. It is a violation of the standard IMRAD (introduction, methods, results, discussion) format to present new data in the discussion section to support an argument you are trying to make. If the data are important enough to be mentioned in the discussion, then these data should be presented in the results.

3.9 Reporting the Number of Enrolled Subjects in the Methods

For studies of human subjects, the methods section should describe the enrollment criteria for study subjects and how the investigators trained study workers to apply these criteria to the community where they implemented the study. The methods section should present the planned sample size and the reason the investigators chose this targeted sample size.

The first sentence of the results should describe how many people were approached, how many agreed to participate, how many were enrolled, and how many had sufficient information collected to be included in the analysis. This opening description of the path to the study population provides the underlying denominator for the subsequent analysis.

The number of enrolled subjects is a topic for the results section rather than methods because there is often some difference between what was planned and what was ultimately implemented. The sample size section in the methods describe the planned sample size. The first line of the results describes the sample size that was ultimately realized.

Examples of the error		Alternative, better options	
✗	In the methods section: "Altogether 330 questionnaires were taken for study."	✓	In the methods section: "Study workers visited the study hospital each morning, approached each inpatient who met the enrollment criteria, and invited them to join the study." In the first sentence of the results section: "Study workers ultimately approached 349 patients meeting the eligibility criteria; 19 refused and 330 completed an interview.

3.10 Specifying the Contents of a Questionnaire

Journals generally limit the number of words in a manuscript. This both saves on paper for printed journals and also helps to preserve the time and attention of readers so that they can focus on the most important elements of the manuscript. With all scientists having more articles to read than they have time, succinct writing improves the influence of your article. Listing the various content area queried within a questionnaire used in the study is neither a good use of precious space nor of the reader's attention. Results from a questionnaire that are relevant to the issues raised in the manuscript will be presented in the results. Readers can infer that this reported information was asked about in the questionnaires. Items that were included in the questionnaire, but are not presented in the manuscript, need not be included in the methods.

By contrast, the physical samples that were collected or the standardized observations that the research team made should be specified.

Examples of the error		Alternative, better options
✗	Between February and March 2014, researchers administered a 45-minute exposure questionnaire among case and control households. The questionnaire collected information about household size, education level, occupation, and age as well as potential exposures related to food consumption, jewelry, kitchenware, housing materials, and farming practices.	✓ Between February and March 2014, researchers administered a 45-minute exposure questionnaire among case and control households.
✗	Field workers collected data using a standardized questionnaire, performed spot checks on hand and domestic hygiene, and collected food samples. **The questionnaires included questions on household sociodemographic factors, household assets, drinking water source, sanitation facilities, food storage duration, food reheating history, and food serving practices.** After the interview was conducted, field workers performed spot checks on food and hand hygiene practices including container types used for cooking and food storage, container cover status, animal presence in the food storage area, feces in the household compound and food storage area, and cleanliness of utensils and mother and child's hands.	✓ After conducting interviews using standardized questionnaires, field workers performed spot checks on food and hand hygiene practices including container types used for cooking and food storage, container cover status, animal presence in the food storage area, feces in the household compound and food storage area, and cleanliness of utensils and mothers' and children's hands.

3.11   Naïve Theories of Change

The underlying motivation for public health research is to generate knowledge that can be used to improve health (in contrast to pure academic research that generates knowledge that is interesting but is not primarily justified by its impact on the world). The introduction section of a public health manuscript explains why the question addressed by the manuscript is important, and the discussion explains the implications of this knowledge. Authors of public health research are expected to explain where their research should lead. This often involves making recommendations that are outside the set of issues where an individual researcher has been professionally trained. When a narrowly trained researcher asserts how to bring about change, the suggestions risk being naïve and therefore not useful. By beginning with a more realistic model of how changes occur, a model of change that is informed with some understanding of history, political science, economics, and sociology, then you can make your scientific work more impactful.

Invoking naïve theories of change create two problems. First, they are lost opportunities. Your published manuscript presents an opportunity to make a credible suggestion to an interested audience on the way forward and to have an impact on public health. A naïve theory of change does not provide useful guidance. Second, naiveté undermines the credibility of your voice, and so of the work, and even of your reputation. Readers conclude, "The author is a narrow scientist who does not understand the world."

3.11.1 Recommending a Massive Increase in Funding

When we evaluate a public health problem in the context of a low-income country and consider how a similar problem is addressed in a high-income country context, it may seem reasonable to ask that local government authorities take the same steps that have been taken in other places to address the problem. The difficulty with this practical sounding advice is that low-income country government authorities do not have access to the same level of funds available to authorities in high-income countries. Failing to appreciate these political and economic constraints is naïve.

Although you are concerned about the specific public health problem that is the focus of your paper, if everyone working on their area of interest always requests the government to provide more money to replicate what high-income countries do, this becomes an impossible agenda for government to fulfil. Indeed, from the perspective of government decision makers, every sector, including transportation, infrastructure, education, economic development, energy, and health, wants more money. While we may passionately believe that allocating more money to the specific problem that is the focus of our research would create a better society, in general, this is not a particularly useful suggestion. The demands on government funds so exceed the available funds that your recommendation is only one among a never-ending chorus of similar requests.

If we cannot make a particular government sector richer, what should we do? As the expert on the topic of the paper you are writing, reflect upon and propose practical suggestions that are cost-effective or, even better, that cost no money or cost less money than is currently being spent to address the issue. Such recommendations are much more likely to be implemented. Identifying practical solutions to problems, or at least pointing out where we can begin to develop practical solutions, is a centrally important way that scientists can improve public health.

3.11.2 Ignoring Incentives and Barriers

Public health studies commonly assess knowledge among residents of low-income countries at risk for a particular health condition. Quite unsurprisingly, such studies generally find that these populations have imperfect knowledge about the health condition under study including ignorance regarding the exposures that increase risk. Many scientific authors then call for an intervention to improve the knowledge of the population and to tell them what they should do.

Such recommendations are naïve because they assume that ignorance is the primary determinant of unhealthy behavior. However, there is abundant evidence both in everyday life and in the scientific literature that knowledge is rarely the primary determinant of behavior. Are people obese because they do not know that eating excessive calorie-dense food leads to weight gain? Do people who smoke cigarettes believe they are using a healthy natural product? Do impoverished households in Bangladesh not serve their children fish more frequently because they are unaware that fish is nutritious?

In general, it is much more productive to consider both the incentives people have and barriers that people must overcome to achieve health rather than a primary focus on improving knowledge. People consume excessive calories for a variety of reasons, including the pleasure of eating, emotional connections to food, and acquired habits. People smoke cigarettes because of addiction to nicotine and enjoyment of the smoking ritual. Poor Bangladeshi households do not eat much fish because they do not have the money to pay for it.

Occasionally, improving knowledge can help to facilitate behavior change, but most knowledge interventions fail to improve health. Thus, when a scientist recommends improving knowledge of the at-risk population as the primary intervention, it suggests to readers that the author is not well read (Error 2.1) and is unaware of the strong and consistent evidence that such knowledge interventions nearly always fail to change behavior. We are much more likely to contribute toward improving health by examining more thoroughly and critically the likely determinants of behavior and then suggesting prevention efforts directed at these determinants.

Example of the error		Alternative, better option
✗	Half of the duck flock owners reported disposing of dead ducks by throwing them into adjacent water bodies. Duck owners should be taught that the Food and Agricultural Organization recommends burying carcasses on site to control avian influenza transmission.	✓ Biosecurity interventions that cost-effectively improve duck survival and egg production are much more likely to be adopted. We recommend further research to develop and evaluate interventions that simultaneously improve duck raisers' profitability and biosecurity.

3.11.3 Assuming Weak States Can Implement

When working on public health problems, we often consider regulatory approaches to constrain unhealthy practices, for example, requiring factories not to discharge toxic pollution into the environment or to have people who provide housing, food, water, education, and health care meet certain standards. Most people expect that some agency within government should maintain and enforce such regulations. Indeed, most people think of such regulations and their enforcement as one of the primary roles of government. Government officials often describe this as being a central part of their role including developing and adopting many such regulations.

However, many governments have limited capacity to enforce such regulations. For example, in rural Bangladesh, Pakistan, Kenya, or Guatemala, do drivers on rural roads routinely obey the speed limits? Do industrial factories routinely treat their emissions so that they meet government standards and do not pollute air or water? In cities, are building codes enforced? Are criminals who commit financial crimes routinely identified tried, convicted, and punished?

Most low-income countries are what political scientists refer to as "weak states." These states have limited capacity across a range of functions, including limited capacity to enforce regulations. Weak states are unable to enforce regulations both because of a lack of technical capacity as well as pervasive incentives that undermine enforcement. Government agencies in weak states lack bureaucratic autonomy [14]. This means that enforcement actions are strongly influenced by political actors. Indeed, some political scientists describe many governments of low-income countries as "predatory states." They argue that such governments exploit their position to extract resources from citizens, without providing the basic functions of government. In weak states, it is relatively easy to pass laws, so it may appear that there is substantial progress, but there is very limited capacity to enforce such laws. There is often no discernible difference in a situation before and after a law is passed.

If authors are working in a weak state but then suggest solutions that presuppose a strong state, for example, Singapore or Germany, perceptive readers conclude that the authors do not understand the context they are working in. This does not improve your credibility as a scientist. Moreover, an approach that requires a strong state will not be effective in a weak state, so the suggestion is not a useful. It does not help move toward a healthier situation. Public health problems generally result from multiple determinants that create an unhealthy situation. Suggesting practical low-cost approaches that can actually improve the situation within the constraints of a low-income context within a weak state is difficult, but this is why deep creativity, hard work, wide reading, conversation with colleagues, and iterative efforts are required tasks of effective public health researchers.

Example of the error		Alternative, better option	
✗	The government of Bangladesh should adopt the manufacturing standards promoted by the European Union to ensure a healthy environment.	✓	Stakeholders responding to incentives have produced the current equilibrium of low-priced bricks with high externalities that harm the environment and health in Bangladesh. Transitioning to an alternative equilibrium that generates less damage to health and the environment will require new approaches that alter the underlying incentives.

3.12   An Insufficiently Focused Introduction

In a standard scientific manuscript, the role of the introduction is very specific: The introduction is not a mini review of interesting themes within the broader field of your study question. The introduction is an argument crafted to persuade the reader of the importance of the study question. An introduction often describes the gap in knowledge that the study addresses and why filling this gap is important for public health or to broaden scientific understanding.

After outlining the introduction, review each assertion and ensure that it directly contributes to a coherent argument that supports the claim that this study question is important. Remove any other points.

Sometimes, understanding the study question requires an explanation of the context of the study or how the present analysis fits within other analyses that have already been published. When this kind of explanation is required so that the reader can understand the relevance and framing of the study question, these elements should also be included in the introduction.

3.13   Failure to Clarify Key Sample Size Assumptions

Estimating a reasonable sample size for a study requires that the researcher predict what the results will be and then apply the laws of probability to calculate the number of observations that would be reasonably expected to demonstrate results of this magnitude with a low probability that observed associations were only due to chance. The most common version of this error is the failure to specify a predicted outcome or the failure to explain why the predicted outcome asserted by the scientist is reasonable.

Scientists do not conduct studies when they already know what the results will be. The argument "I don't know what the outcome is; that is why I am conducting this study" is not an acceptable reason for the absence of a defensible argument for sample size. If it were an acceptable argument, it would apply to all studies. Estimating a sample size is an exercise similar to developing a budget for an activity. We cannot foresee all expenses, but we make a judgment based on prior experience to estimate the costs. Similarly, when calculating sample size, we make an estimate of what we think we will find and explain why we think so. Perhaps there will be studies from other regions that have looked at this phenomenon or a similar phenomenon. Alternatively, you may argue that unless a problem is of a certain magnitude, then either it is not important enough or we accept that we won't have sufficient power to see it. A funding agency will look at the sample size estimate and ask if the money they are investing is likely to achieve the study objectives. They do not want to overpay, but they want reassurance that their money will not be wasted because the sample size was too small to reach the objectives.

A common variation on this error occurs when the primary study outcome is prevalence. The scientist predicts that the outcome will be 50% because they read in a statistics textbook that estimates near 50% require the largest sample size and so they want to be maximally conservative. This is unreasonable because calculating sample size requires an estimate both of the outcome variable and a reasonable level of precision. If the estimated prevalence is 50%, then a study that estimates this prevalence $\pm5\%$ may be reasonable. By contrast, if the estimated prevalence is 3 per 10,000, then assuming an estimated prevalence of 50% $\pm5\%$ would generate a proposed sample size that is far too low.

There is no simple statistical rule that allows a scientist to assert a sample size by a mechanical process that bypasses estimating an outcome and making a reasoned argument for this judgment. When writing a manuscript, the methods section should clarify the assumptions that the scientists originally made of the study outcomes.

Examples of the error	Alternative, better options
✗ We calculated a sample size of 400 based on 80% power and 95% confidence.	✓ We assumed, based on studies of indoor air pollution from cooking (Alam NE 2004, Jones FJ 1997), that children living in a village located within one kilometer of a brick kiln would be at 30% increased risk of pneumonia compared with children who live in villages > 5 kilometers from a brick kiln. We assumed an incidence of pneumonia in this community would be 45 per 100 child years of observation (SE Arifeen 2007), so a sample size of 400 would provide 80% power to detect a difference in groups of 30% at 95% confidence.
✗ We assume that 50% of the poultry workers (~380) will experience at least one episode of symptomatic illness during the study period.	✓ An earlier study found that 44% of adults in an urban community in Dhaka developed a symptomatic episode of influenza-like illness between March and September (MA Azziz 2006). We assumed that 44% of poultry workers would experience at least one episode of influenza-like illness during 6 months of observations.

3.14 A High-Level Outline That Is Not High Level

The objective of a high-level outline is to sketch out the major components of the manuscript that will support the data analysis included in the framing document (see 1.2.2). The phrase "high level" means that the document outlines the major issues for the manuscript, not all of the details or even all of the components that will be included in the manuscript. The narrative should be no longer than 1500 words; 1200 words is even better.

If your narrative outline is longer than 1500 words, respect the time of your co-authors, and edit it to focus on key ideas prior to sharing it. Bullet points are fine. This is not the time for refining grammar and English language scientific prose.

3.15   Specifying Software Used for Routine Data Analysis

There are innumerable elements that contribute to a study that supports a scientific manuscript, but the manuscript need not, indeed cannot, specify all of these elements. For example, it is not necessary to mention the brand and version of word processing software that was used to craft the study protocol. It is not necessary to specify the email program that the principal investigator used to communicate with co-investigators or the operating system that was used on the data server. Similarly, if the statistical analysis is routine, the name of the software program used for data analysis need not be specified. Routine analysis includes calculations of means, medians, standard deviations, interquartile ranges, prevalence, incidence, odds ratios, prevalence ratios, risk ratios and their accompanying 95% confidence intervals, simple linear regression, multiple linear regression, and multiple logistic regression.

The underlying guiding principle for writing the methods section is that the methods should be presented in sufficient detail so that other investigators could replicate the study. If the statistical calculations are routine, they could be conducted on any available statistical platform. However, if the researchers used a nonstandard approach that perhaps required special programming in R or a module that is available only in a particular software package, but is not widely available, then it is appropriate to specify the software and procedure that was used. If not, don't squander the readers' limited attention with this irrelevant detail.

In the interest of improving validity and reproducibility, more and more journals are requiring scientists to make the primary data and their analytical code publicly available. There are several platforms including the Open Science Framework (https://osf.io/) that permit this. When posting the analytical program used to analyze the data, it is important to characterize the analytical software and the version number within the posting though it need not be mentioned in the manuscript.

Examples of the error		Alternative, better options	
✗	We performed descriptive statistics using STATA version 14 software.	✓	~~We performed descriptive statistics using STATA version 14 software.~~
✗	We conducted all of our analysis using R version 3.1.0.	✓	Our prespecified analysis plan is available (https://osf.io/6u7cn/).

3.16   Presenting Rationale in the Last Sentence of the Introduction

In a standard public health or biomedical manuscript, the last sentence of the introduction is a succinct statement of the objective of the manuscript. All of the other text in the introduction is basically an argument on why the objective is important. When an author inserts a sentence or two after the statement of objectives and concludes with a rationale, this confuses the reader because the basic narrative form has been violated. It makes it difficult for someone who is scanning a paper to quickly identify the objective.

Examples of the error	Alternative, better options
✗ This study aimed to identify national-level menstrual hygiene management knowledge and practices among adolescent school girls and facilities provided by their schools. We examine the association of menstrual hygiene management knowledge, practice, and school facilities with absence from school during menstruation. Findings from this study can guide Bangladesh government policy on female education and inform future initiatives to increase female student attendance and school performance.	✓ This study aimed to identify national-level menstrual hygiene management knowledge and practices among adolescent school girls and facilities provided by their schools. We examine the association of menstrual hygiene management knowledge, practice, and school facilities with absence from school during menstruation. ~~Findings from this study can guide Bangladesh government policy on female education and inform future initiatives to increase female student attendance and school performance.~~

The rationale is an important aspect of the introduction (see Error 3.12). It is simply out of place at the end of the introduction.

Articles published in economic journals are an exception to this rule. In an economics journal, the last sentence of the introduction explains the organization of the paper.

Open Access   This chapter is licensed under the terms of the Creative Commons Attribution 4.0 International License (http://creativecommons.org/licenses/by/4.0/), which permits use, sharing, adaptation, distribution and reproduction in any medium or format, as long as you give appropriate credit to the original author(s) and the source, provide a link to the Creative Commons license and indicate if changes were made.

The images or other third party material in this chapter are included in the chapter's Creative Commons license, unless indicated otherwise in a credit line to the material. If material is not included in the chapter's Creative Commons license and your intended use is not permitted by statutory regulation or exceeds the permitted use, you will need to obtain permission directly from the copyright holder.

Chapter 4
Mechanics of Writing

4.1 Using Nonstandard Acronyms

A great barrier to communication is overuse of TLAs. When you work on a specific topic, you become quite comfortable with a TLA. You make it up or hear others in your project or area use it, and pretty soon, you are using it. When the time comes to write, instead of using words that people understand, you use TLAs throughout your manuscript. A TLA is a three-letter acronym. An acronym is a type of abbreviation where a new word is formed from the first letters of a series of words. It is annoying to read a passage that is written in code.

While acronyms have meaning to those who use them every day, as soon as a document is shared with outsiders, acronyms become an obstacle to understanding. Using acronyms requires readers to learn a new vocabulary. Indeed, scientific authors commonly expect readers to learn several new complex multisyllabic phrases simply to understand the article. Most people do not learn new language quickly. A reader may need to go back to the manuscript and review how the acronym was defined. Perhaps the reader highlights the acronym in another color so they can more quickly decode the work. Asking the reader to exert cognitive attention to try to learn and remember a new acronym leaves less attention available to the substance of the manuscript. Readers may skip over the acronyms or guess what they mean from context because they do not have the time or inclination to go back through the manuscript and figure out what it stands for.

Writers often assume that readers are similar to themselves. This is a flawed assumption. It is best to avoid all acronyms all the time. Using the replace feature of any word processor, you can remove them from your text. This means more people can understand your writing, including, for example, journal editors and journalists who are not topic experts in your area and staff who work for policy makers. An article that can be understood without decoding will be understood by more people. A more understandable article is more likely to influence global understanding.

© The Author(s) 2022
S. Luby, D. L. Southern, *The Pathway to Publishing: A Guide to Quantitative Writing in the Health Sciences*, https://doi.org/10.1007/978-3-030-98175-4_4

Authors demonstrate respect for readers by avoiding insider abbreviations. Using words removes the burden from readers of requiring them to refer back to the first use of the abbreviation to decode meaning.

When journalists report on scientific work, they rarely use acronyms. Why not? Because they are experts in textual communication. They want people to understand what they write.

The few exceptions to this rule pertain to acronyms that are so standard that the general population would understand them (e.g., HIV, CDC). However, even for these, the acronym should be spelt out the first time it is used in the manuscript. The Editor of the American Journal of Public Health states this succinctly, "We frown on all acronyms but those in universal use." The editors of the American Journal of Tropical Medicine and Hygiene maintain, "Abbreviations are commonly overused, compromising the clarity of manuscripts. Authors are advised to keep abbreviations to a minimum, using them when they are clearer than long terms (e.g., PCR, DNA), but avoiding them when possible when they are non-standard and idiosyncratic." The "Uniform Requirements for Manuscripts submitted to Biomedical Journals" (www.icmje.org) recommends, "Avoid abbreviations in the title and the abstract."

Examples of the error		Alternative, better options	
✗	The NTCP has not been evaluated.	✓	The National Tuberculosis Control Program has not been evaluated.
✗	The CSF is scheduled to begin at 12 noon every Monday.	✓	The Centre for Scientific Forum is scheduled to begin at 12 noon every Monday.

4.2   Using Nonstandard Spaces

This error is particularly common among authors who draft their manuscripts using justified alignment where the text falls flush on both the right and left margin rather than left justification (Error 4.8). All the squeezing and spreading of spaces required by justification makes it more difficult for the author to detect spacing errors.

You can avoid irritating reviewers and journal editors with this distracting error by checking your document before sending it. Use the "Find and Replace" feature of your word processer. Search for two spaces and replace them with one. If you click on the replace all button, this removes all the double spaces in the document. You may have to repeat this process a couple of times if you also have some triple or larger series of spaces within your document. If you take this simple step after you spell-check and before circulating the document, then you can consistently avoid this error.

Nonstandard spacing includes:

1. The absence or too many spaces before or after parentheses.

Example: *To evaluate compliance with current World Health Organization(WHO) guidelines of postexposure rabies treatment(PET), we interviewed all animal bite victims. One-hundred-nine(76%) bites were category III and 33(23%) were category II.*

This is incorrect. There should be a space after "Organization" and before "(WHO)." Similarly, there should be a space after 'treatment" and before "(PET)". There should be a space after "nine" and before "(76%)." There should be a space after "33" and before "(23%)."

2. The absence of spaces following a comma.

Example: *On average the workers completed five household interviews,three child assessment,and one structured observation per day.*
This is incorrect. There should be a space after the word interviews and after the word assessment.

3. Inserting more than one space between words.

Example: *Approximately 6 million people annually undergo postexposure treatments worldwide, most in Third World states as a consequence of failure of canine rabies control programs or strategies.*
This is incorrect. There should be only one space after the word *"undergo"* and only one space after the word *"as."* There should also be one space between sentences, not two.

4. Inserting a space within a numeral > 1,000

Example: Field workers collected samples from 12, 456 patients.
This is incorrect. There should be no space after the comma (Error 4.11). The numeral should be written as 12,456.

4.3   Improper Spelling

Improper spelling is distracting and unnecessary with the advent of spell-checking. Be sure to thoroughly spell-check any document you ask others to review.
    Some journals prefer British English spelling. Others prefer US spelling. Set the spell-checker in your word processor to be consistent with the spelling specified in the Instructions to Authors for your target journal. If the Instructions to Authors does not specify a preference, review recent published articles from the journal to see what they use. Use the spell-checker to align spelling for the narrative elements of the manuscripts. Also check titles, legends, and contents of figures and tables. However, do not change the spelling in references or in the proper names of institutions.

Example of the error		Alternative, better option	
✗	Mixture of United States English and United Kingdom English	✓	Harmonize spelling in article to meet the requirement of the journal.
✗	Centres for Disease Control and Prevention	✓	Centers for Disease Control and Prevention

4.4 Capitalization Problems

4.4.1 Using All Capital Letters

Look at an article in your target journal. Is the title of the article written in all capital letters? Are the titles of the tables and figures in all capitals? Are the words that are column and row headings in all capitals?

The reason that portions of journal articles are not written in all capitals is that reading text that is written in all capital letters is annoying. Indeed, research has demonstrated that people read all capital letters more slowly than they read standard sentence case. Thus, prepare your draft in accordance with the standards of the literature.

To learn more, navigate to Google Scholar (http://scholar.google.com/). Input the search terms "Reading speed all capitals," and review the nearly 100-year history of research demonstrating the reduced readability of all capital lettering.

Take a lesson from the clarity of scientific findings. Avoid all capitals. If you want to emphasize a title or a heading, use a larger font or **bold.**

4.4.2 Capitalizing Non-proper Nouns

Although you may commonly use the acronym IEC to refer to information, education, and communication, that does not make these words proper nouns requiring capitalization. A proper noun refers to a specific person or place. Barak Obama and the Director General of Health are proper nouns requiring capitalization but not acquired immune deficiency syndrome (AIDS).

Example of the error	Alternative, better option
✗ In low-income countries, Information, Education, and Communication (IEC) should focus on high-risk sexual behavior.	✓ In low-income countries, information, education, and communication should focus on high-risk sexual behavior.

4.5 Failure to Spell Out an Isolated Numeral < 10

The International Committee of Medical Journal Editors (www.icmje.org) used to suggest that numbers < 10 should be spelled out in the text ("four" instead of 4). However, since 2010, they no longer make this recommendation. Different journals have different preferences on this issue. Unless journal copy editors recommend otherwise, we recommend you present numerals if you have a direct comparison or multiple numbers in a sentence, some less than ten and some more than ten, but write out numbers less than ten if they stand alone.

Example of the error		Alternative, better option	
✗	The field team identified 6 community residents with fever and mental status changes.	✓	The field team identified six community residents with fever and mental status changes.
✗	Following the intervention, five of the 45 health centers were observed to have adequate practices.	✓	Following the intervention, 5 of the 45 health centers were observed to have adequate practices.

4.6   Starting a Sentence with a Numeral

Example: 43 individuals (56%) tested positive to more than one dengue serotype. 24 of them were reactive to type 1 and 2.

Historically, many journal and copy editors have considered this incorrect and not permitted it. Others argue that we should present numbers so they can be easily assimilated and compared. Trying to compare a number that is spelled out in English to a number that is numerically presented in the same sentence is an unnecessary chore—much like trying to read material that is in all capitals.

If you look in leading scientific journals, for example, *Lancet* and *Science,* you can find examples of articles with numerals beginning a sentence and numerals less than 10 presented numerically.

What should a writer do? The first goal of a writer is to provide clarity and quick understanding. If it is reasonable to initiate a sentence with a number, then do so. If editors do not permit it, then alternative strategies include:

- Write out the numeral in words.
- Recast the sentence so that it doesn't begin with a numeral though be careful not to make the sentence too awkward.
- String sentences together with semicolons because the next word following a semicolon does not need to be capitalized; thus, numerals are permitted.

Examples of the error		Alternative options	
✗	50 respondents did not complete the survey.	✓	Fifty respondents did not complete the survey.
✗	24 study participants (45%) correctly recalled the health education message that they had received.	✓	Of the respondents, 24 study participants (45%) correctly recalled the health education message that they had received.
✗	43 (56%) individuals tested positive to more than one dengue serotype. 24 of them were reactive to type 1 and 2.	✓	Forty-three individuals (56%) tested positive to more than one dengue serotype; 24 were reactive to type 1 and 2.

4.7   Not Indenting Paragraphs

To make it clearer to your readers, how your paper is organized into different ideas and/or sections, it is important to indicate when one paragraph ends and when another begins. The standard format is to indent the first word of each paragraph one tab width (0.25–0.5 inch).

An alternative form is to skip a line between paragraphs. If you do skip a line between paragraphs, it is still best to indent the first word. This way, when a new page starts with a new sentence, it is clear to the reader whether or not this also starts a new paragraph.

4.8   Not Aligning Text to the Left

Setting your word processor so that it aligns text to both the left and right margin (justify) distorts the space between letters and makes it more difficult for the reader to read the text. Although it creates a clean look along the left and right side of the page, it makes it difficult to identify spacing errors. Leave such text alignment to the journal that will finally format your article. For drafts that you send for review, you want to make these as easy on your co-authors and reviewers as possible. Align all text to the left.

4.9   Problems with Parentheses

Using parenthetical phrasing to qualify statements with additional verbiage should be avoided in the narrative portion of a manuscript. If you initially draft a sentence that deploys parenthetical clarification or qualification, consider revising the sentence to communicate your ideas without parentheses. This allows the reader to understand your ideas without backtracking and revising their understanding of your meaning.

1. Using parentheses to clarify language.

Incorrect example: *Personal harm (physical injury) of a friend was reported by 10%.*
Alternative: *Ten percent of students reported that a friend was physically injured.*
Incorrect example: Most (but not all) respondents agreed that the community benefited from the new water pump.
Alternative: Seventy-five percent of respondents agreed that the community benefited from the new water pump.
Incorrect example: *Children whose parents were employed in an informal industry (e.g., garbage picking, lead acid battery recycling, brick manufacturing) were*

less likely to be immunized against measles than children whose parents owned their own business or were employed in the formal sector.

Alternative: *30% of parents were employed in informal industries including garbage picking, lead acid batter recycling, and brick manufacturing. Children whose parents were employed in an informal industry were less likely to be immunized against measles than children whose parents owned their own business or were employed in the formal sector.*

2. Putting numbers and percentages in parentheses.

Parentheses are helpful in adding specific numbers to support a narrative claim.

Incorrect examples:

The majority (64, 92%) of women reported associated symptoms.

Correct examples:

The majority (n=64, 92%) of women reported associated symptoms.
The majority (64, [92%]) of women reported associated symptoms.
Women were 2.2 times (95% confidence interval 1.8, 2.6) more likely to develop illness than men.

4.10 Not Recognizing When an Abbreviation Has Become a Name

Institutions often begin with one name, but as they evolve, the original name no longer describes the institution and so the name changes. For example, AT&T used to be the American Telephone and Telegraph Company. IBM used to be International Business Machines. BRAC used to be the Bangladesh Rural Assistance Committee. Sometimes, institutions have an official name (Leland Stanford Junior University), but a different name that the institution actually uses as its regular name and brand (Stanford University).

The acronym for the International Centre for Diarrhoeal Disease Research, Bangladesh, was a communications nightmare: It was neither simple nor easy to understand. It failed to accurately describe what the institution did. Beginning in 2010, the institution rebranded and, like AT&T and BRAC, now wants its former acronym to be its formal name, icddr,b. Note that with this rebranding, the institution's name is not capitalized.

Journal editors or reviewers will often assume that icddr,b is an acronym (as it was in the past) and request that it be in all capital letters and spelled out. When responding to this request, it may be helpful to use examples of other acronyms that have become names, for example, AT&T, IBM, or BRAC.

4.11   Misplaced Commas in Large Numbers

The standard placement of commas in numbers greater than 999 in international communication is with a comma after every three digits from the right and no spaces between digits or between the comma and the digits. The comma is optional, but it can be particularly helpful to readers to understand numbers especially when they exceed five digits. The placement of commas and the use of spaces are often different in the Asian subcontinent, but for scientific writing, or anytime you are writing for an international audience, large numbers should be recorded in standard international form.

Examples of the error		Alternative, better options	
✗	7, 51,842	✓	751,842
✗	51, 00,000 doses of vaccine	✓	5,100,000 doses of vaccine

4.12   Varying Fonts Within the Narrative

The font used for narrative text of the manuscript should be a consistent size and style. If the first paragraph is Times New Roman 12 point, then so should each of the subsequent paragraphs. Sometimes during copying, pasting, or other editing variable, font sizes or types are introduced. Consistency avoids distracting the reader.

Examples of the error:		Alternative, better options:	
✗	We randomly divided consented households into two groups. Fieldworkers visited Group A each Sunday and Wednesday and visited Group B on Tuesdays and Thursdays.	✓	We randomly divided consented households into two groups. Fieldworkers visited Group A each Sunday and Wednesday and visited Group B on Tuesdays and Thursdays.
✗	We randomly divided consented households into two groups. Fieldworkers visited Group A each Sunday and Wednesday and visited Group B on Tuesdays and Thursdays.	✓	We randomly divided consented households into two groups. Fieldworkers visited Group A each Sunday and Wednesday and visited Group B on Tuesdays and Thursdays.

4.13   Using Bulleted Lists Rather Than Sentences

A list of phrases or words with preceding bullets works well for outlining, for quickly communicating a list on a website summary, or, if not overused, on slides that accompany an oral presentation. Although we are quite accustomed to communicating ideas in this format, this is not the standard technique for communicating in a scientific manuscript. Scientific manuscripts use sentences that flow together in paragraphs. There is a long history of written English language that uses sentences and paragraphs. Indeed, the complexity and nuance that characterizes scientific ideas makes this traditional format work quite well. Moreover, it is what editors and readers expect.

Examples of the error		Alternative, better options	
✗	The field team also conducted spot checks to observe the following: • Latrine status (hygienic or unhygienic) • Presence of open feces (both human and animal) within the courtyard • Raw food remnants (food waste produced during food preparation) or leftover food within the courtyard • Food storage practices	✓	The field team also conducted spot checks within the household compound to observe the type and cleanliness of the latrine(s), presence of animal or human feces and food waste within the courtyard, and food storage practices.
✗	The defining features of all of these permutations of a District-Based Approach to intervening in the water and sanitation sector are: • A commitment by an intervening organization to work for a period of time longer than that needed for single projects within a specific subnational administrative district, such as a municipality or county (but smaller than a state or equivalent) • Sets a goal of achieving universal access to water and sanitation services within that district • Explicitly working with the local government • Develop capacity in the local government/public sector for planning and maintaining water and sanitation services • Align with the country's national water and sanitation policy, while engaging, to varying degrees, with national government	✓	The defining features of the district-based approach appear to include an institutional commitment to work long term in a specific subnational administrative district, a goal of achieving universal access to water and sanitation services within that district, explicitly working with the local government, and alignment with the country's national water policy while engaging.

4.14   Uninformative Document Names

The scientific document that you create will be shared with your co-authors, many of whom are likely to be co-authors on many other scientific documents. It helps your co-authors and reviewers keep track of your work if you create names for your document that are specific. The clearest document names include a description of the document and a version number. It also can be helpful to include your name and possibly a date.

Examples of the error	Alternative, better options
✗ Manuscript.docx	✓ Simple Soap Man v13.docx
✗ Review response.doc	✓ Response to Ecohealth Reviewers v3.doc
✗ Concept note.docx	✓ Detecting_lead_in_spices_Concept_note_Jenna v2.docx

Open Access   This chapter is licensed under the terms of the Creative Commons Attribution 4.0 International License (http://creativecommons.org/licenses/by/4.0/), which permits use, sharing, adaptation, distribution and reproduction in any medium or format, as long as you give appropriate credit to the original author(s) and the source, provide a link to the Creative Commons license and indicate if changes were made.

The images or other third party material in this chapter are included in the chapter's Creative Commons license, unless indicated otherwise in a credit line to the material. If material is not included in the chapter's Creative Commons license and your intended use is not permitted by statutory regulation or exceeds the permitted use, you will need to obtain permission directly from the copyright holder.

Chapter 5
Grammatical Structures and Stylistic Strategies

5.1 Using Present Rather Than Past Tense

When your work is published, it becomes a historical document. Years, even decades, later, people can look back at what you did at that time in that place and what you learned. The present tense might sound OK to your ear as you are writing your first draft and the project is still ongoing, but after 1 or 2 years elapses before your manuscript appears in print, and another couple of years before a reader pulls it out of a MEDLINE search, the present tense will not be correct.

Editors will insist on the past tense, so from the beginning, draft your paper in the past tense. Present tense can only be used in the introduction or the discussion to report established facts, for example, "Tuberculosis is a leading cause of death among adults in low-income countries."

Similarly, avoid using words that imply a timeliness, such as currently, recently, lately, or in the past year. When referring to conditions at the time of writing or the time of observation, specify the month and a year. In an ongoing outbreak or pandemic, when you want to share the latest time-bound data, keep updating the figures in your subsequent drafts. Just before you submit your paper to a journal, update the figures. Do the same when resubmitting after the peer review.

Examples of the error		Alternative, better options	
✗	We enroll every fourth house as part of our study.	✓	We enrolled every fourth house as part of our study.
✗	Data derived from the Thatta Health System Research Project are used for the study.	✓	We used data derived from the Thatta Health System Research Project for the study.
✗	Currently, the total number of lab-confirmed cases has increased to 3,167 cases with 583 deaths.	✓	In June 2021, the total number of lab-confirmed cases was 3,167 cases with 583 deaths.

© The Author(s) 2022
S. Luby, D. L. Southern, *The Pathway to Publishing: A Guide to Quantitative Writing in the Health Sciences*, https://doi.org/10.1007/978-3-030-98175-4_5

5.2   Failure to Use Definite and Indefinite Articles

What is an article? An article modifies a noun. English has two articles: **the** and **a/an**.

Neither Bengali, the language of Bangladesh and West Bengal, nor Urdu, the most common language spoken in Pakistan, use definite or indefinite articles. Speakers whose first language does not use articles do not have an intuitive pattern to apply to English.

The is a definite article. It is used to refer to specific or particular nouns. For example, if I say, "Let's read **the** book," I mean a *specific* book.

A/an are indefinite articles. Indefinite articles modify nonspecific or nonparticular nouns. For example, if I say, "Let's read **a** book," I mean *any* book rather than a specific book. If I say, "I would like to go see **an** art exhibit," I don't have a *specific* art exhibit in mind. There are many art exhibits, and we could be talking about *any* art exhibit. The indefinite article **a** is used when the next word begins with a consonant (e.g., a paper, a writer). The indefinite article **an** is used when the next word begins with a vowel (e.g., an article, an author).

A specific error commonly made by scientific writers for whom English is a second language and whose first language does not use articles is using the word "majority" without a preceding article. Whenever you use the word "majority" in your scientific writing, ensure that an article precedes it.

Examples of the error		Alternative, better options	
✗	Majority of cases (83%) took advice, while very few (17%) did not consult anybody.	✓	The majority of cases (83%) took advice, while very few (17%) did not consult anybody.
✗	We reviewed the hospital logbook to determine in which subdistricts majority of patients resided.	✓	We reviewed the hospital logbook to determine in which subdistricts the majority of patients resided.
✗	Majority of respondents thought the new design was an improvement.	✓	A majority of respondents thought the new design was an improvement.

5.3   Excessive Use of Passive Voice

With active voice, the subject does the action of the verb.
Active voice example: The *study team administered a questionnaire.*

The study team is the subject. The subject performed the action that is administered the questionnaire.

In passive voice, the subject is acted upon. It does not actively perform the verb. The subject is passive.

Passive voice example: *A questionnaire was administered.*

The questionnaire did not do the action of the verb. The questionnaire did not administer. It was acted upon by the verb. It was administered.

In general, writing should be composed in the active voice because of the immediacy and precision conveyed when the subject of the sentence carries out the action.

Active voice is more efficient than passive voice. It takes the reader from point A to point B in a "straight line." Active voice usually requires fewer words. It communicates who the actor was and so provides more specificity. Active voice is closer to normal conversational speech and usually reads easier and with greater clarity. In other areas of writing, for example, business writing and journalism, active voice is almost universally preferred.

Although passive voice is used in many scientific articles, especially in the methods section, active voice is increasingly common. Although some writers use passive voice to convey the appearance of an objective, fact-based discourse, not limited to or biased by individual perspectives or personal interests, its imprecisions risks conveying that the authors are unwilling to specify who took the action.

If you are willing to use the word "we," your manuscript will be more readable. If you can communicate the same idea in active voice or in passive voice, choose active voice. Your text is likely to have more impact.

When to Use Passive Voice   It is not always an error to use passive voice. Passive voice is particularly useful, even recommended, in two situations:

1. When it is more important to draw our attention to the person or thing acted upon

Correct passive example: The results of the study will be published in the next issue of the journal.
Instead of writing: *The editor of the journal will publish the results of the study in the next issue.*

2. When the actor in the situation is not important: Passive voice is especially helpful in scientific or technical writing or laboratory reports where the process or principle being described is of ultimate importance.

Correct passive example: *The first coat of primer paint was applied immediately after the acid rinse.*
Instead of writing: *The first author applied the first coat of primer paint immediately after the acid rinse.*

Examples of the error		Alternative, better options
✗	A non-inferiority analysis was done.	✓ We conducted a non-inferiority analysis.
✗	A sample was selected.	✓ We selected a sample.
✗	Questionnaires were administered to the household head.	✓ Fieldworkers administered the questionnaire to the household head.

5.4   Improper Use of "We"

A major advantage of using active voice is that it specifies who did the action. It is important that this attribution of action be correct. A manuscript's authors collectively write the manuscript. When the manuscript uses the word "we," this refers to the authors. Work that is conducted by fieldworkers or other members of the team who are not on the author line should not be attributed to the authors.

Examples of the error		Alternative, better options	
✗	We revisited households 3 and 6 months after receiving the filter to assess usage.	✓	Fieldworkers revisited households 3 and 6 months after receiving the filter to assess usage.
✗	We interviewed households at baseline and weekly from August 2005 to September 2006.	✓	Trained enumerators interviewed households at baseline and weekly from August 2005 to September 2006.

5.5   Writing from a Psychological Perspective

Science assumes that the external world, the world outside of our minds, is real. Scientific articles describe observations of this external world and attempts to integrate them into larger theoretical understanding. What interests or surprises people varies and often depends upon their personal experiences and their affection for particular hypotheses or transient fads that are quite unrelated from careful inference drawn from scientific observations. Thus, when you write emails to your family or articles for the popular press, you can include subjective considerations, for example, interests, surprises, and shock. However, when you are writing a scientific manuscript, you should focus on the ideas relevant to the issues examined in your study and the consistency of ideas and theories with available evidence.

Examples of the error		Alternative, better options	
✗	We were surprised to find that people admitted to using alcohol in a country where its use is restricted.	✓	Although alcohol sales and consumption are officially prohibited in the country, 30% of respondents reported drinking alcohol in the preceding month.
✗	The incremental cost of adding *Haemophilus influenza* type B vaccine to the existing immunization schedules in low-income countries may not be as high as imagined.	✓	Adding *Haemophilus influenza* type B vaccine to the existing immunization schedules in low-income countries would increase the national immunization budget by 4%.

5.6   Using Excessive Subheadings in the Discussion

For most articles presenting original research in most journals, the discussion section (unlike the methods section) is not subdivided. In standard manuscript format, a section explaining limitations and a section drawing conclusions are included in the discussion section as outlined in Appendix 6. These sections should not have a separate header labeled "limitations," "recommendations," or "conclusions" unless the journal you are preparing the article for has a specific requirement for such a section.

An exception to this rule applies when a long discussion that engages two or three separate themes is easier for readers to understand if these themes are called out separately. Only use this approach if you confirm that articles published in your target journal use subheadings in the discussion.

5.7   Misplaced Modifiers

A misplaced modifier is a word or phrase that is meant to modify one object in a sentence, but its placement in the sentence implies that it modifies a different object. Sometimes, the reader can figure out what the author meant; other times, the meaning is ambiguous. Even if the reader can figure out the meaning, it is sloppy grammar that risks distracting readers.

Examples of the error		Alternative, better options	
✗	Interventions to reduce the risk of pig-related diseases can compromise the social and economic situation of pig raisers in predominately Muslim countries who may already be stigmatized.	✓	Interventions to reduce the risk of pig-related diseases in predominately Muslim countries can compromise the social and economic situation of pig raisers who may already be stigmatized.
✗	Then field staff selected four girls from each school for interview who had reached menarche.	✓	Then field staff selected four girls who had reached menarche from each school to interview.
✗	Since 2006, surveillance physicians maintained a registry of patients admitted to three Nipah surveillance hospitals meeting the encephalitis case definition: fever or history of fever with axillary temperature >38.5°C (101.3°F) with altered mental status, new onset of seizures, or new neurological deficit.	✓	Since 2006, surveillance physicians at the three Nipah surveillance hospitals maintained a registry of admitted patients who met the encephalitis case definition: fever or history of fever with axillary temperature >38.5°C (101.3°F) with altered mental status, new onset of seizures, or new neurological deficit.

5.8   Using Nouns with Awkward Syntax in Place of Verbs

English is a flexible language. By adding a suffix, the same root word can often function as either a verb or a noun. At times, however, this flexibility generates awkward, complex constructions. Communication is optimized by succinct clear language.

Examples of the error		Alternative, better options	
✗	Community members exhibited a preference for open defecation.	✓	Community members preferred defecating in the open.
✗	The dominant advice for zoonotic spillover prevention is a reduction in direct physical contact with nonhuman primates.	✓	The dominant advice to prevent zoonotic spillover is to reduce direct physical contact with nonhuman primates.
✗	This useless equipment represents a genuine harm to health-care facilities in low-income countries.	✓	This useless equipment harms health-care facilities in low-income countries.

5.9 Using Different Terms for the Same Object or the Same Idea

To avoid mind-numbing repetition, authors commonly vary word choice and style throughout the manuscript. Although such variation can engage readers, if it is applied to scientific terms, it risks confusing readers.

Examples of the error		Alternative, better options:	
✗	Using "injuries" in one sentence, "accidents" in another sentence and "wounds" in a table.	✓	Define the term injury as "damage inflicted on the body by an external force" in the methods section. Use the term injury consistently throughout the manuscript.
✗	Using "birds" in one sentence, "poultry" in another sentence and "chickens" in a table.	✓	Define the term poultry as "domesticated fowl raised for meat or eggs." Only use the term bird or chicken if you intend a different meaning.

Open Access This chapter is licensed under the terms of the Creative Commons Attribution 4.0 International License (http://creativecommons.org/licenses/by/4.0/), which permits use, sharing, adaptation, distribution and reproduction in any medium or format, as long as you give appropriate credit to the original author(s) and the source, provide a link to the Creative Commons license and indicate if changes were made.

The images or other third party material in this chapter are included in the chapter's Creative Commons license, unless indicated otherwise in a credit line to the material. If material is not included in the chapter's Creative Commons license and your intended use is not permitted by statutory regulation or exceeds the permitted use, you will need to obtain permission directly from the copyright holder.

Chapter 6
Achieving Clarity and Conciseness

6.1 Labeling Rather Than Explaining

We love our technical terms. We've studied them; we learn them, and now while writing a manuscript, we finally have a chance to use them! Right? Well, actually not.

Labeling is shorthand for the full development of an idea, but people often have a different idea of exactly what that shorthand actually means. The same term often carries different meaning to people with different disciplinary backgrounds. This makes using these terms a barrier to clear communication.

Strive to explain exactly what you did. Do not label it. The more specific you are about exactly what you did, the easier it is for someone else to understand it. If a methods section reads, "For the hospital catchment area survey, we selected 20 unions, using a probability proportional to size sampling approach," a reader may wonder, What is a probability proportional to size sampling approach? How did you apply this concept to your site? The methods section should report methods in sufficient detail so that other investigators could repeat them. So skip the label, and instead use the space to describe the steps you took to identify and enroll the population.

The three most common labeling issues in papers concern study design, sampling methods, and limitations.

Examples of the error		Alternative, better options	
✗	The population of the catchment area was projected for 2008 on the basis of the 2001 Bangladesh census using population estimation by component method.	✓	We began with the 2001 Bangladesh census of subdistrict populations and applied national estimates of crude birth rate, net external migration, and national crude death rate (ref) to estimate the population in the subdistricts at the time of the assessment.

© The Author(s) 2022

S. Luby, D. L. Southern, *The Pathway to Publishing: A Guide to Quantitative Writing in the Health Sciences*, https://doi.org/10.1007/978-3-030-98175-4_6

Examples of the error	Alternative, better options
✗ Confounding by wealth is a potential limitation.	✓ Households who had windows that provided cross ventilation may have been wealthier and possessed other characteristics that improved their children's health that we were unable to completely control for in the analysis.

6.2   Using Weak Opening Phrases for Sentences

You should try to use phrases and transitions that advance the ideas and arguments of the paper. By contrast, most of the phrases below reflect the psychological state of either the reader or the writer. Strive to write from the perspective of the ideas you are developing. You are better off having no transition than using such vacuous phrases as the examples below:

Examples of the error		Alternative, better options
✗	It was found out that...	✓ *Delete*
✗	One important observation from the findings of this study was that...	✓ *Delete*
✗	We conclude from our data...	✓ *Delete*
✗	Moreover, our survey showed that...	✓ *Delete*
✗	Therefore, this will not be an overstatement that...	✓ *Delete*
✗	It is known that...	✓ *Delete*
✗	It can be seen from the above table that...	✓ *Describe*
✗	The explanation could be that...	✓ *Explain*

6.3   Using Adjectives and Qualifiers

Adjectives are words that modify a noun. Adjectives often imply substantial subjective and emotional content, both of which should be minimized in conventional scientific writing. For example, what is "important" or "large" to one person may not be "important" or "large" to another.

Qualifiers are words that modify an adjective, but do not carry a specific meaning, such as "very." The addition of a qualifier adds to the subjectivity, as in "very important." It is better to try to choose the best adjective, and provide justification of its use, and not to use a qualifier.

Examples of the error	Alternative, better options
✗ The outbreak caused very high mortality.	✓ 56% (301/536) of people infected in the outbreak died.
✗ This very large outbreak.	✓ This outbreak affected 300 school children.

Examples of the error		Alternative, better options	
✗	The incidence was much higher in children <5.	✓	The incidence among children <5 was six times higher than older children.

6.4   Overusing Studies or Authors as Sentence Subjects

In general, when referring to other scientific work, the subject of the sentence should not be the study, or the study's author, but the core ideas or results that connect to your manuscript. Ideas and observations referenced from other studies are central to scientific reasoning. The use of a study or a study's author as the subject of a sentence risks distracting the reader from the substance that links to the author's own study. The structure of your sentences should reflect this prioritization of ideas and results over individuals and authors.

Example of the error		Alternative, better option	
✗	A study by Yoruba in Tanzania suggested that 78% of the clients who presented to traditional healers were females, 95% of whom were illiterate and of a low socioeconomic group (ref).	✓	Demographic parameters are important because they may influence health-seeking behavior; a study in Tanzania, for example, found that educated mothers are more likely to discourage traditional healing practices (ref).
✗	Curtis et al. have championed structured observation as the preferred approach to measuring handwashing (ref).	✓	Using structured observation to assess handwashing behavior has consistently identified lower frequencies of handwashing with soap compared with reported behaviors.

6.5   Using Nondescriptive Numeric or Alphabetical Labels

Study teams commonly develop some study-specific vocabulary, for example, Group A and Group B and Phase 1 and Phase 2. The study team becomes so familiar with these labels and their underlying characteristics that they use these labels in everyday conversation within the study team. Unsurprisingly, when team members start writing about the study, they commonly use these same labels.

However, such labels are inappropriate for a scientific document intended for readers outside of the study team. Such nondescriptive numeric or alphabetic labels require readers to learn the study team's private code, or not be quite sure what all the differences reported by encoded classification actually represent. The team's private code is broadly useless information not applicable to any other manuscript the reader will ever encounter. Avoid needlessly frittering away your readers' attention. Make your paper as easy to understand as possible. Use descriptive labels for each group.

This is particularly important when constructing figures. Figures should clearly label groups being compared without requiring the reader to go back into the methods section or other aspects of the paper to decode the key characteristics that distinguish the groups.

Examples of the error		Alternative, better options
✗	At baseline, group 1 participants were somewhat less likely to own a television than group 2.	✓ At baseline, participants enrolled from Tongi were less likely to own a television than participants enrolled from Narshindi.
✗	Compared with baseline, contraceptive prevalence increased by 12% in phase 1 and by another 10% in phase 2.	✓ Compared with baseline, contraceptive prevalence increased by 12% after steps to improve supplies in clinics and by another 10% after community outreach.
✗	Category A symptoms included cough and difficulty breathing, while category B symptoms included diarrhea and vomiting.	✓ Respiratory symptoms included cough and difficulty breathing. Gastrointestinal symptoms included diarrhea and vomiting.

6.6 Using Respectively

The word "respectively" is an adverb meaning "in the order given." Although it is commonly deployed in scientific writing to summarize results in few words, it is best avoided. A sentence ending with "respectively" requires the reader to go backward, reread, and mentally connect words and numbers that are physically disparate on the page. This extra effort risks interrupting the reader's engagement with the flow of your manuscript's narrative. Strive to make your sentences easy to read and understand without backtracking.

Examples of the error		Alternative, better options
✗	Of the plasmodium-positive children, 17 (4%) and 9 (2%) were positive for *P. falciparum* and *P. vivax,* respectively.	✓ Of the smear-positive children, 17 (4%) had *P. falciparum* and 9 (2%) had *P. vivax.*
✗	Attack rates for any postoperative infection between the suspected outbreak period January and December 1996 and for comparison period June and December 1995 were 14% (10/72) and 6% (2/31), respectively.	✓ The attack rate for any postoperative infection between the suspected outbreak period January to December 1996 was 14% (10/72) compared with 6% (2/31) between June and December 1995.
✗	Household size differed in rural, peri-urban, and urban communities with a mean of 6.4, 4.2, and 3.2 members, respectively.	✓ Mean household size differed in rural (6.4), peri-urban (4.2), and urban (3.2) communities.

6.7   Using the Word Etcetera

Scientific writing is characterized by precision. "Etcetera" is not specific. This imprecision suggests that the author's ideas have not been fully formulated or have not been fully thought through. "Etcetera" should never appear in a scientific concept paper, protocol, or manuscript.

Example of the error		Alternative, better option	
✗	Medical costs in the hospital included admission fees, bed rent, diagnostic tests, medicine, consultation fees, etc. Nonmedical costs included travel, food, tips, etc.	✓	Medical costs in the hospital included admission fees, bed rent, diagnostic tests, medicine, and consultation fees. Nonmedical costs included travel, food, and tips.

6.8   Using a Non-English Word as an English Word

Most scientific articles aim for international readership. Words and expressions that are specific to the country where the work was conducted risk confusing international readers. In English language scientific articles, words from other languages should be *italicized and placed in parenthesis.*

Example of the error		Alternative, better option	
✗	We conducted a case-control study in two upazilas in Rajshahi district.	✓	We conducted a case-control study in two subdistricts (*upazilas*) in Rajshahi district.
✗	Anthropologists interviewed gaccis in each village.	✓	Anthropologists interviewed date palm sap collectors (*gaccis*) in each village.
✗	The questionnaire was translated into Bangla.	✓	The questionnaire was translated into Bengali. *Note: Bangla* is not an English word. The English language word for the language spoken in Bangladesh is Bengali (not italicized). When writing about questionnaires in Latin America, scientists do not use the Spanish word for the Spanish language (*español*). They do not write that the questionnaires were translated into *español*. Instead, they write that the questionnaires were translated into Spanish. Similarly, when writing in English about work in Bangladesh, we should refer to the local language as Bengali.

6.9   Describing Costs Only in Local Currency

International readers of scientific manuscripts are unlikely to be familiar with the value of local currency. They will have difficulty interpreting costs described in local currency.

The US dollar is the most widely used currency globally and so provides a useful metric to communicate cost to international readers. Importantly, many scientific articles aim to reach both an international scientific audience and a local audience, and so it may be useful to present costs in both currencies.

At a minimum, include an appropriate conversion (the one prevailing at the time data was collected) between the local currency and an international currency so that readers can connect the currency in your paper to amounts of money they understand.

Examples of the error		Alternative, better options	
✗	The mean monthly household income in the study communities was 4916 Pakistan rupees.	✓	The mean monthly household income in the study communities was US$ 370 (4916 Pakistan rupees).
✗	The cost per fully treated patient at a government hospital in Mexico City was 3200 MXN.	✓	The cost per fully treated patient at a government hospital in Mexico City was US$ 162 (3200 MXN). *Note:* In the methods section include the exchange rate (1 US$ = 19.8 Mexican pesos (MXN) and the date the currency was converted on (June 7, 2021).

6.10   Using the Term "Developing Country"

The term "developing country" is nonstandard and imprecise. All countries are developing. Belgium was a different country in 2020 than it was in 2000. It had a higher income and a greater number of internet connections. It was developing. Belgium will look different in 2044 than it did in 2020. It will develop further. Although the term "developing" historically connotes industrial development, there is no standard definition that can be consistently applied to classify countries as a "developing country" or not.

By contrast, the World Bank has clear standards for characterizing countries by income level. It assigns the world's economies to four income groups—low, lower-middle, upper-middle, and high-income countries. The classifications are updated each year on July 1 based on gross national income (GNI) per capita in current USD (using the World Bank Atlas method exchange rates) of the previous year.

6.11   Using the Term "Socioeconomic Status" as a Synonym for Wealth

When referring to income or poverty/wealth among persons, households, or communities, many writers mistakenly use the term socioeconomic status. If the available measurements are strictly measurements of wealth or income, for example, household assets, then use terms that refer to this narrower concept. For example, wealth, income, or poverty level. Socioeconomic status and wealth are not synonyms. The concept of socioeconomic status captures more than just wealth. It encompasses income, education, and profession and also includes the idea of social class. Restrict the use of the term socioeconomic status only when the available data supports this broader conceptualization.

6.12   Using a Technical Term in Its Nontechnical Sense

Several technical scientific terms carry a less specific meaning when used in general speech. To avoid confusing the reader, avoid using technical terms in their nontechnical sense.

6.12.1   Using the Term "Random" in Its Nontechnical Sense

The term "random" has a specific technical meaning within science. Random selection, for example, implies that the entire population is enumerated and that a process, such as a lottery or a random number generator, is used to select individuals from among the entire population. In a scientific manuscript, the word "random" should only be used within this specific context.

In common speech, the word "random" is often used as a synonym for "haphazard." For example, "I was walking down the street and selected a restaurant for lunch at random." To a scientist, this was not random selection of a restaurant. Rather, the choice of lunch location was based on convenience.

Example of the error	Alternative, better option
✗ In-depth interviews were conducted with 10 randomly selected key informants working in health centers.	✓ We conducted in-depth interviews among 10 key informants we identified who worked in health centers in the study communities.

6.12.2   Using the Term "Reliable" in Its Nontechnical Sense

The term "reliable" has a specific technical scientific meaning that is narrower than its meaning in common speech. Within science, "reliability" refers to whether repeated measurements of the same phenomenon are similar. A blood test is reliable if it provides the same result on repeated testing of the same sample. The synonym for "reliability" in this technical sense is "repeatability." To avoid confusing your scientific reader, the words "reliable" and "reliability" should only be used in their strict technical sense in any scientific document.

Example of the error		Alternative, better option	
✗	The self-reported data may not be reliable.	✓	The self-reported data may not be valid.
✗	The direct observations were conducted to cross-check the responses and ensure reliability of the data collected in the self-administered survey.	✓	We cross-checked the findings from the self-administered survey by comparing them with results from direct observation.

6.12.3   Using the Term "Significant" in Its Nontechnical Sense

The term "significance" has a specific technical meaning in quantitative scientific writing. Specifically, it refers to statistical associations that are less likely than would be expected by chance. Conventionally, these are associations with a probability of occurring by chance of less than 5%. Many thoughtful commentators on scientific writing are critical of this narrow dichotomous conceptualization that divides all results into "significant" or "not significant" (see Error 7.1.1). Despite this criticism, when scientific readers see the term "significant" in a scientific manuscript, they will assume the author is referring to statistical significance. Avoid using the term in a different context or you risk confusing the reader.

Example of the error		Alternative, better option	
✗	A significant number of respondents could not identify common signs of H5N1 in poultry (Table 2).	✓	Most respondents could not identify common signs of H5N1 in poultry (Table 2).
✗	Backyard poultry can be a significant source of high-quality protein for rural low-income families.	✓	Backyard poultry can be an important source of high-quality protein for rural low-income families.

6.12.4   Using the Term "Valid" in Its Nontechnical Sense

The term "valid" has two related technical meanings in quantitative scientific writing. When used to describe a measurement, it implies that the measurement reflects the underlying phenomenon of interest and is not an artifact of the instrument being used for measurement or other cause of inaccuracy.

When used to describe a scientific inference, the term valid implies that the inference is sound given the results and the way the data were collected. The term is used more loosely in general communication. To avoid confusing readers in scientific manuscripts, only use the term in its technical sense.

Example of the error		Alternative, better option	
✗	Preventing nosocomial transmission of tuberculosis is especially valid in Bangladesh because of its high tuberculosis burden.	✓	Preventing nosocomial transmission of tuberculosis is important in Bangladesh because of its high tuberculosis burden.
✗	The similarity of results from the repeated assessment of the samples suggests that the assay is valid.	✓	The similarity of results from the repeated assessment of the samples suggests that the assay is reliable.

6.12.5   Using the Term "Incidence" Incorrectly

Epidemiologists define incidence as the number of new cases of illness that occur in a specified population in a specified time. For example, the incidence of hepatitis B in the population was 23 cases per 10,000 persons per year. The numerator for incidence is a count of new cases (or new events). The denominator is person-time, that is, a measure that captures both population size and time. Because time is in the denominator, incidence is always a rate. Thus, the second word of the phrase "incidence rate" is redundant.

Prevalence, by contrast, is the number of cases in a population. It includes both new cases and old cases. For example, there may be 400 cases of hepatitis B in the same population of 10,000 people. Most of these cases are old cases. The prevalence of hepatitis B in the population is 4%.

Reporting incidence as an unqualified percentage is incorrect because it does not communicate the time frame that the new cases occurred.

Example of the error		Alternative, better option	
✗	We followed a cohort of live poultry market workers in Bangladesh to determine the seroprevalence and incidence rate of seroconversion of antibodies to H5N1 virus.	✓	We followed a cohort of live poultry market workers in Bangladesh to determine the seroprevalence and incidence of seroconversion of antibodies to H5N1 virus.
✗	The incidence of diabetes among Marin County residents, 5%, is the lowest in the state.	✓	The prevalence of diabetes among Marin County residents, 5%, is the lowest in the state.

6.12.6   Using the Term "Correlated" Incorrectly

In statistics, the term "correlated" implies that there is a statistical relationship between two continuous variables. In common speech, the term correlation often implies any sort of statistical association. In scientific writing, only use correlated when it is technically accurate.

Example of the error		Alternative, better option	
✗	Cross-sectional quantitative studies have found that higher trust was correlated with increased compliance with Ebola control measures.	✓	Cross-sectional quantitative studies have found that higher trust was associated with increased compliance with Ebola control measures.
✗	Consistent correlations were noted between ethnicity and a variety of health outcomes.	✓	Ethnicity was associated with a variety of health outcomes.

6.13   Using the Term "Documented"

The word "document" is a noun. English often turns nouns into verbs, but not always with good results. To "document" means to make a document, that is, to write something down. So if you write down on a piece of paper the phrase "the earth is flat," then, strictly speaking, you have documented that the earth is flat. Creating a document is unrelated to the validity of an assertion. Therefore, we should not use this verb to communicate scientific validity of a statement.

Example of the error		Alternative, better option	
✗	Studies in Bangladesh, India, and Malaysia also documented neutralizing antibodies against Nipah virus in *Pteropus* bats.	✓	Studies in Bangladesh, India, and Malaysia also identified neutralizing antibodies against Nipah virus in *Pteropus* bats.

6.14   Framing an Argument in Terms of Need

Quite often, arguments in draft scientific papers are framed in terms of needs. The underlying message is that we "need" to do something. Usually, the authors are asking the reader, the government, or society more generally to care about the issue in the same way that the authors care about the issue and follow the specific advice of the authors.

In a scientific manuscript, it is reasonable to talk about a need for water, oxygen, and food for survival, but it is less appropriate to assert a need for health-care reform or a need for social change. The problem with this language is that it disguises the goals and aspirations of the authors in terms of a need when the issue of what constitutes a legitimate need is an open question for individuals, for society, and for science.

Scientific writing is most persuasive when it demonstrates the connection between a set of conditions and consequences. Rather than framing arguments in terms of needs, the same ideas should be described as steps that are required to achieve a particular outcome. Importantly, the outcome should be specifically stated.

Examples of the error		Alternative, better options	
✗	There is a need to standardize and expedite the assignment of causes of death, thereby enhancing a timely process of appropriate decision-making.	✓	If the assignment of causes of death could be standardized, appropriate decision-making based on these data could be expedited.
✗	A low-cost, accurate approach to characterize handwashing behavior is needed.	✓	A low-cost, accurate approach to characterize handwashing behavior would improve the assessment of handwashing promotion programs.

6.15   Using the Term "Illiterate" as a Synonym for "No Formal Education"

Although we often use the word "illiterate" as a synonym for "no formal education," these terms are not synonymous. Literacy can be evaluated by asking people if they can read or write and validated using specific literacy tests. People may have attended school for some years and still not be able to read or write. People who have not attended formal schooling are unlikely to be able to read and write, but it is more precise to characterize their lack of education rather than their literacy skills. The term illiterate also sometimes carries a condescending tone and so risks communicating a lack of respect for one's study subjects.

Examples of the error		Alternative, better options	
✗	The age range of program beneficiaries was 18–65 years old, and over 25% who took part in activities were illiterate.	✓	The age range of program beneficiaries was 18–65 years old, and over 25% who took part in activities had less than 4 years of schooling.
✗	Educated mothers were 2.3 times more likely to have a handwashing station with soap and water than illiterate mothers.	✓	Educated mothers were 2.3 times more likely to have a handwashing station with soap and water than those with no schooling.

6.16   Using the Word "Challenging" as a Synonym for "Difficult"

We often use the word difficult to describe public health problems or solutions. The word is appropriate as major problems are characteristically complex and defy simple solutions. The word challenging is often used as a synonym for difficult, but challenging carries a different connotation. The root noun of the adjective challenging is challenge. The connotation is that the situation is testing us; that by engaging in this issue our capacity to take on new issues and to grow to address these issues is revealed. When a situation is difficult, motivational coaches encourage us to see this difficulty as a personal challenge so that we can strive to overcome it.

This implicit motivational jargon is out of place in scientific writing that values precise description. The substitution of challenging as a synonym for difficult is so overused that it risks sounding insincere. If the situation is difficult, then call it difficult. If you want to challenge a group, in an editorial or in the discussion section, then do so explicitly.

Examples of the error		Alternative, better options	
✗	We will explore challenges in implementation, as well as find out what factors motivate children to participate.	✓	We will explore difficulties in implementation, as well as find out what factors motivate children to participate.
✗	In these impoverished contexts, changing child feeding behavior is challenging.	✓	Poverty is a major barrier to improving child-feeding behavior.
✗	These modest findings highlight the challenges of maintaining high-quality implementation of interventions at scale.	✓	These modest findings highlight the difficulties of maintaining high-quality implementation of interventions at scale.

6.17   Describing a Laboratory Test Result as Positive

Scientific communication is characterized by specificity and nuance. It avoids unqualified generalizations. Scientific thinking eschews narrow dichotomies, such as stating that an intervention was a success or failure. Instead, a scientific approach is more likely to identify aspects that achieved objectives and aspects that did not.

Scientific writing should bring this framing to our description of laboratory results. No laboratory test is 100% sensitive and 100% specific. A laboratory test provides additional information that scientists can interpret. When describing laboratory results, use sufficiently precise language so that readers can interpret the meaning without having to jump back to the methods section to review which laboratory tests were conducted and how they were interpreted.

Examples of the error		Alternative, better options	
✗	Out of 23 samples tested for different respiratory viruses, 21 were positive for respiratory syncytial virus.	✓	Out of 23 samples tested for different respiratory viruses, 21 had detectable RNA for respiratory syncytial virus.
✗	From the surveillance database, we identified 209 influenza-positive patients during May to October 2010.	✓	From the surveillance database, we identified 209 laboratory-confirmed influenza patients during May to October 2010.
✗	Among the 123 people tested, six were positive for Nipah.	✓	Among the 123 people tested, six had IgM antibodies against Nipah virus.

6.18 Using Increase or Decrease in the Absence of a Time Trend

The words increase or decrease imply a change in quantity over time. They should not be used when comparing two groups during the same time interval.

Example of the error		Alternative, better option	
✗	Children < 5 had an increased risk of infection compared with school-aged children.	✓	Children < 5 had a higher risk of infection compared with school-aged children.
✗	Children in the nutrition intervention group had a decreased prevalence of anemia compared with controls.	✓	Children in the nutrition intervention group were less likely to have anemia than controls.

The words increase and decrease can be used appropriately when evolution over time has occurred. For example, the incidence of anemia decreased between 2003 and 2015.

6.19 Describing a Test as a Gold Standard

The phrase "gold standard" has a precise meaning in economic history, but this overused phrase is too imprecise for scientific communication. Most commonly, authors use it in a context when a laboratory test yields few false positives. However, in many situations, the errors generated by false-negative tests are as equally misleading and harmful as false-positive tests.

The term "gold standard test" implies an argument from authority that the authors used the best test. Arguments of authority are received skeptically by scientists (Error 2.3.3). All tests have advantages and disadvantages. All tests require thoughtful interpretation. When discussing the use of a specific test or a comparison between two tests, communication is improved by specifying the particular characteristics that are being compared and contrasted.

Example of the error		Alternative, better option	
✗	Enteric fever surveillance is often based on blood culture, the current gold standard diagnostic test for enteric fever.	✓	Enteric fever surveillance is often based on blood culture because the absence of false-positive results provides confidence that each identified case is a confirmed case.
✗	We compared the seroprevalence of the total reported positive tests in the area to understand the level of underreporting from gold standard RT-PCR testing.	✓	We compared the seroprevalence of IgG antibodies against SARS-CoV-2 to the government reports of respiratory specimens from residents of these communities who had SARS-CoV-2 RNA detected by RT-PCR testing.

Open Access   This chapter is licensed under the terms of the Creative Commons Attribution 4.0 International License (http://creativecommons.org/licenses/by/4.0/), which permits use, sharing, adaptation, distribution and reproduction in any medium or format, as long as you give appropriate credit to the original author(s) and the source, provide a link to the Creative Commons license and indicate if changes were made.

The images or other third party material in this chapter are included in the chapter's Creative Commons license, unless indicated otherwise in a credit line to the material. If material is not included in the chapter's Creative Commons license and your intended use is not permitted by statutory regulation or exceeds the permitted use, you will need to obtain permission directly from the copyright holder.

Chapter 7
Recording Scientific Data

7.1 Using Statistics in Place of the Study Question to Frame Results

We become so enamored with the output of our statistical programs and our statistical understanding that sometimes our narrative reads like the output of our statistical analysis program. You know you are making this mistake when words like "association," "analysis," or "relationship" are the subject of a sentence or when the name of variables used to code the data appears in the manuscript.

The point of analysis of health data is not mathematical output but what these results mean in terms of the lives and health of people. The results should be expressed and communicated with other health professionals in terms of the research question.

Examples of the error		Alternative, better options	
✗	Father's literacy was associated with immunization status (p=.007).	✓	Children whose fathers were educated were more likely to be completely immunized than children of uneducated fathers (84% versus 44%, p =.007).
✗	In simple regression analysis, education and pregnancy status give highly significant relationship, while language and counseled by give significant relationship on screening.	✓	Women who were educated, who spoke Hindi, and who benefited from counseling from a physician were more likely to consent to the screening test.
✗	The analysis of association among the independent variables showed that there is an association between the main exposure variable (Distgrp2) and the costgrp and between costgrp and the duration of disease (Durdgrp2).	✓	People who lived farther from health facilities spent more money per visit to the health-care facility.

© The Author(s) 2022
S. Luby, D. L. Southern, *The Pathway to Publishing: A Guide to Quantitative Writing in the Health Sciences*, https://doi.org/10.1007/978-3-030-98175-4_7

7.1.1 Framing Narrative Results Around P-Values

A p-value assesses the probability that results as extreme as observed in the analyzed groups could have arisen by chance enrollment of a nonrepresentative study population. Scientific authors should assess how likely chance is a credible explanation for observed differences, but a p-value < 0.05 does not prove an association is causal. It does not provide insight on whether the association is due to bias. It does not assess whether the association is due to confounding.

A low p-value conflates whether an association between exposure and outcome have a large effect (which may have quite important impacts on the scientific or public health implications of the results) or whether there is a small or even trivial effect in a large number of observations. (If the sample size is one million, all of the p-values will be <0.001.)

As the authors of a formal assessment of the use of p-values in biomedical literature noted, "p-values do not provide a direct estimate of how likely a result is true or of how likely the null hypothesis is ('there is no effect') true. Moreover, they do not convey whether a result is clinically or biologically significant. P-values depend not only on the data but also on the statistical method used, the assumptions made, and the appropriateness of these assumptions" [15].

In short, p-values are silent on most important dimensions of assessing valid scientific inference. Presentations of results should not be framed around p-values. Indeed, framing results around p-values communicates to the reader that the author has a naïve approach to data interpretation. Instead, frame results around effect sizes and presenting work in an order so that readers can consider issues of confounding, bias, and dose effect and present p-values like a footnote, not as a central finding. Think of "statistical significance" as only an issue of second-order concern, that is, if there is a difference that is potentially meaningful and interesting, it provides a test of whether this difference is likely due to chance selection of a nonrepresentative study population.

Framing a scientific narrative around p-values also encourages a naïve dichotomous conceptuality, that is, that a factor is either present or absent. Science is characterized less by this sort of absolute binary frames and more about measuring degrees of difference.

The editors of the *International Journal of Epidemiology* explain their perspective on this issue. "We actively discourage use of the term 'statistically significant' or just 'significant' and statements in method sections such as 'findings at p<0.05 were considered significant.' Where used, we ask authors to provide effect estimates with confidence intervals and exact P values, and to refrain from the use of the term 'significant' in either the results or discussion section of their papers. Our justification of this position is given in Sterne J, Davey-Smith G. 'Sifting the evidence – What's wrong with significance tests?' *BMJ* 2001: 322:226-231."

Examples of the error		Alternative, better options	
✗	When we looked at the contamination of each toy ball separately, two toys did not reach statistical significance for fecal coliform contamination.	✓	When we compared fecal coliform contamination between groups for each toy ball separately, toys were consistently less contaminated in the cleaner households compared to the less clean households. However, the comparison between groups of fecal coliform contamination of toys 2 and 4 did not reach statistical significance (Table 2).
✗	Compared with persons who contracted Nipah infection from another person, Nipah cases who drank raw date palm sap were more likely to develop convulsion (log rank p-value <0.001), altered mental status (log rank p-value <0.001), and die (log rank p-value <0.001).	✓	Compared with persons who contracted Nipah infection from another person, Nipah cases who drank raw date palm sap were three times more likely to develop convulsions, 50% more likely to develop altered mental status, and 58% more likely to die (log rank p-values all <0.001).

7.2   Not Presenting the Core Data

Your most engaged readers are not only interested in your conclusions. They want to look at the data and draw their own conclusions. This is the essence of science-reflective consideration of empiric observations. Your manuscript should present the data in a way that allows the reader to form an independent opinion as to whether the data were analyzed properly and interpreted prudently. As a matter of transparency, the reader should be able to redo the key calculations. Thus, basic frequencies, rates, or means comparing groups on your central findings are crucial.

A common variant of this error occurs when comparison between groups is limited to measures of association or percentages without the underlying numbers. In its most extreme form, the measure of association is omitted entirely. Only a p-value is presented (see Error 7.1.1).

Examples of the error		Alternative, better options	
✗	Most subjects (62%) were not aware of ….	✓	Of 113 subjects, 70 (62%) were not aware of…. *[always show numerators and denominators in the calculation of proportions.]*
✗	There was a significant difference in the proportion of case-patients and control-subjects who reported eating the potato salad (p=0.0001).	✓	Of the 42 case-patients, 30 (71%) reported eating the potato salad compared with 19 of the 120 control-subjects (16%, odds ratio=13.3 p<0.01).
✗	Proportions only in the tables	✓	Always provide numerators and denominators.

7.3   Using Too Many Decimal Places

When the results of a study are presented with an excessive number of decimals, communication between the writer and the reader is impaired. The extra digits distract the reader from the message. Presenting too many decimal places also implies a precision that the data generally lack.

This error is most commonly seen with percentages. Data are presented as percentages, for example, 39%, rather than as frequencies, for example, 321/815, so that it is easier to remember and compare one group or scenario to another. Although 10,000 decimal places are a more precise report of the percentage, it is burdensome for the reader. For example, if 13 of 17 enrolled study subjects have a particular characteristic, this can be reported as 76%, 76.5%, 76.47%, 76.461%, 76.46706.... With a powerful enough calculating program, you could report thousands or millions of decimal places.

However, reported percentages with multiple decimal places are no longer easy to remember and compare. Active readers who want to understand the meaning of your scientific writing will often compare reported numbers to each other. It is much easier for readers to compare numbers and to perform mental arithmetic on rounded numbers. Thus, wherever possible, note percentages without decimal places. Only include decimals if the percentage is less than 10, and the figures beyond the decimal point have public health significance.

Similarly, when people report relative risk or confidence intervals, they often report it to two decimal places, for example, the statement that people who ate goat curry were three times more likely to become ill than persons who did not (relative risk of 3.24, 95% confidence interval CI=0.74–12.99, p value=.143). Can your investigation reliably estimate the relative risk and the confidence interval to two decimal places? If the study cannot support such precision, then you should not imply that level of precision by reporting the extra decimal places.

One rule of thumb for confidence intervals for odds ratio is that they should not have more than two meaningful figures. Whether or not these figures are decimals or not depends upon where the odds ratio fit on a log scale. Remember that the odds ratios for "protective exposures" and "risk factors" are symmetrical around the number one on a log scale. Thus, reporting an odds ratio of 243 represents the same amount of precision as an odds ratio of 24.3, an odds ratio of 2.43, and an odds ratio of 0.243. Thus, try to round up (add or subtract digits) so that you always display two meaningful figures, for example, 24, 2.4, or .24.

Examples of the error		Alternative, better options	
✗	The prevalence of active trachoma was 21.01% (95% confidence interval: 6.23–36.77%).	✓	The prevalence of active trachoma was 21% (95% confidence interval: 6.2–37%).
✗	People who ate goat curry were three times more likely to become ill than persons who did not (relative risk of 3.24, 95% confidence interval CI=0.74–12.99, p-value=0.143).	✓	People who ate goat curry were three times more likely to become ill than persons who did not (relative risk of 3.2, 95% confidence interval CI=0.74–13, p-value=0.15).

7.4   Using Too Few Decimal Places

In the enthusiasm to avoid using too many decimal places, occasionally, authors present too few. In most contexts, you want to communicate two digits of numerical information (25% is two digits. $1.2 million is two digits). As noted in 7.3 reporting, a percentage greater than 10, adding a third digit, a decimal place, is generally distracting and uninformative. However, if you are reporting an odds ratio or other relevant small number, then it is important to communicate two digits of information (2.1 or 0.63) even if one or more of these digits are decimal places. Count digits, not decimal places!

Examples of the error		Alternative, better options	
✗	Children whose mother completed primary education were less likely to be hospitalized for diarrhea (odds ratio 0.6, 95% confidence interval 0.4, 0.8).	✓	Children whose mother completed primary education were less likely to be hospitalized for diarrhea (odds ratio 0.57, 95% confidence interval 0.42, 0.77).
✗	Ambulatory case-patients spent a median of US$2 (IQR=$1–4) in the public hospitals.	✓	Ambulatory case-patients spent a median of US$1.8 (IQR=$1.1–3.6) in the public hospitals.

7.5   Using Incomplete Headings for Tables and Figures

In a biomedical manuscript, the figures and tables should stand alone. A reader should be able to look at the table or figure, read the title, and understand it. Readers should not have to refer to the narrative methods or results to understand the table or the figures. Thus, a typical heading reporting on a study population should include person, place, and time. The number of study subjects and statistical methodology should be communicated. Use footnotes to explain apparent discrepancies or other issues in the table/figure that benefit from further clarification.

Tables and figures that are developed for slides to accompany verbal presentations are different than tables developed for manuscripts. Slide visuals are designed to be understood quickly. Brief titles for tables and figures in these slides are preferred.

Examples of the error		Alternative, better options:	
✗	Figure 1: Epicurve of the measles outbreak	✓	Figure 1: Cases of measles by date of onset, Chennai City, Tamil Nadu, November 2004
✗	Table 2: Risk factors associated with illness, univariate analysis	✓	Table 2: Characteristics of meningitis case-patients and control subjects, Kano City, Nigeria, March 1996

7.6   Imbalance Between Table and Narrative Presentation of Results

7.6.1   Too Little Narrative Explaining the Tables

Just as tables, figures, and graphs should stand on their own and not require accompanying text, the narrative section of the results should stand alone. A reader should be able to read only the narrative text, not look at any of the figures or tables, and come away with a clear understanding of the important findings from the analysis. This error most commonly takes the form of several well-constructed tables being presented in the results section with only a sentence or two in the narrative results section pointing to each table. The results section should not repeat all the data that is in a table but rather should focus the reader on the highlights. Look at several quality journal articles related to your research question, and note the balance between what is presented in the narrative text and what is presented in the tables. Strive for a similar balance.

Example of the error		Alternative, better option	
✗	Of all the food items, only the vanilla ice cream was associated with illness (Table X).	✓	The risk of illness was estimated according to consumption of each of the eight menu items that were served at the lunch (Table X). Eating vanilla ice cream was the only exposure that was significantly associated with illness (relative risk: 8.6, p=0.001) and that accounted for the majority of cases (population attributable fraction: 86%).

7.6.2   Too Much Narrative Explaining the Tables

Some manuscripts deploy excessive narrative to comment on nearly every number presented in a table. This includes reiterating minor findings that are not relevant to the core issues engaged by the manuscript. A key responsibility of the analyst is to reduce data so it is more easily understandable to the reader. The narrative results section of a manuscript should summarize the primary findings and highlight findings that contribute importantly to the interpretation of the results. Avoid overrepetition of data that is more easily seen and compared in a well-constructed table.

7.6.3   Presenting Results in Narrative that Would Be Clearer in a Table

Comparison of a few numbers can be clearly understood when presented in a narrative paragraph, but when there are many numbers, subgroups, and comparisons, a table is a more efficient format for communication. Tables allow the readers to quickly compare columns and subgroups and so understand the relationships among all of the observations.

Examples of the error	
✗	A total of 4046 blood cultures were performed from study participants hospitalized in the inpatient department of Hospital A (n=2363) and Hospital B (n=1683). Of these, 694 (17%) were positive for *Salmonella* Typhi or Paratyphi. 421 (18%) of blood cultures from inpatients in Hospital A and 208 (12%) in Hospital B grew *S.* Typhi, while 39 (2%) of blood cultures from inpatients in Hospital A and 26 (2%) in Hospital B grew *S.* paratyphi.
	A total of 4046 blood cultures were performed from study participants enrolled as outpatients department of Hospital A (n=6225) and Hospital B (n=5094). Of these, 694 (6%) were positive for *Salmonella* Typhi or Paratyphi. 435 (7%) of blood cultures from outpatients in Hospital A and 208 (12%) in Hospital B grew *S.* Typhi, while 10 (0.2%) of blood cultures from outpatients in Hospital A and 14 (0.2%) in Hospital B grew *S.* paratyphi.

Alternative, better option						
✓			Tested	*Salmonella* typhi		*Salmonella* paratyphi
				No.	%	No.	%
	Hospital A						
	Inpatient		2363	421	18%	39	2%
	Outpatient		6225	435	7%	10	0.2%
	Hospital B						
	Inpatient		1683	208	12%	26	2%
	Outpatient		5094	289	6%	14	0.3%
	Total		**15365**	**1353**		**89**	

7.7   Pointing Too Explicitly to Tables and Figures

In your results section, if the words "Table 1" or "'Figure 2" are the subject of a sentence, you have likely committed this error. The paper should be organized around the central ideas you want to communicate and that you want the reader to focus on. Thus, lead with your findings, and compose your language around those findings and related ideas rather than around structures, that is, pages, tables, or figures.

Examples of the error		Alternative, better options	
✗	Table 1 describes the forms in which areca nut was used.	✓	Sweetened varieties of areca nut were the most popular (Table 1).
✗	Figure 2 presents the age, sex, and geographic distribution of our sample across the four study districts.	✓	The age, sex, and geographical distribution of the samples was similar across the four study districts (Figure 2).

7.8   Using Inappropriate Figures

Edward Tufte, in his excellent book, *"The Visual Display of Quantitative Information,"* argues that figures for scientific manuscripts should be evaluated using a data to ink ratio. He urges communicating the most data with the least ink. Excessive ink in figures mean they include unnecessary axes, grid lines, borders, 3-D effects, and other elements that do not add substance and make the figures less understandable.

Space is at a premium for print journal editors, who weigh this issue more from the perspective of data to space ratio. Both pie charts and simple frequencies presented as bar charts are inefficient. It is reasonable to assume that the reader of a scientific manuscript understands the difference between 20% and 40% and so does not need it illustrated by comparing relative widths of a pie or relative heights of a bar. A simple table can efficiently present proportions.

Thus, use figures to achieve key communication objectives. Figures are best used in two situations:

1. When they permit presenting a large amount of data in a format that reveals the underlying characteristics of the distribution, for example, scatter plots that show trends
2. When they communicate in a more effective and efficient visual format than can be achieved with a narrative description or a table, for example, a figure that presents multiple components of a phenomenon, such as different age trends by sex, or presents the data in a way that reveals an important relationship

7.9   Generic Data Tables That Lack a Clear Message

There is no single standard format to present data in tables. Tables are an integral element of the broad scientific argument that you compose through your manuscript. Tables should be organized based on the communication objective of the article. Thus, the first step in drafting a table is to identify the communication objective for the table. Examples might be to describe the baseline characteristics of the population, to compare the outcome of a group who received an intervention with the outcome in a nonintervention group, or to compare the characteristics and exposures of persons who became ill with persons who remained well.

First, specify the communication objective of the table. Then construct the table so that the message comes through clearly. The patterns in the data that you are striving to illustrate should be obvious at a glance or at least should be obvious once they have been pointed out by the narrative description in the results section of the manuscript [16]. Just like narrative scientific writing, expect to develop and revise tables through several drafts.

7.10   Table Layout That Impairs Comparisons

An advantage of presenting data in tables, rather than in a narrative paragraph, is that by clearly aligning numbers, different groups and different characteristics can be readily compared. Numbers are easier to compare reading down columns than across rows especially for larger numbers of items. Such comparisons are often the central communication objective of a table. To facilitate comparison, avoid:

- Columns that are too wide. This makes it difficult to compare data between columns. One common form of this error is to set the width of the table column based on the length of the column heading rather than on optimizing column width to permit comparison of data.
- Ordering data haphazardly. Rather than presenting characteristics in the table in alphabetical order, or in the order they were asked in the questionnaire, consider the easiest way for the reader to understand the information. Ordering characteristics from smallest to largest or largest to smallest is an intuitive approach that helps the reader to quickly and easily understand.
- Poorly aligned data that impedes comparison. Align data and decimals so that a vertical list is readily comparable.

Hard to compare	Easier	Still Easier
23 42 34 109 87 42 27 98 114 75	23	23
	42	27
	34	34
	109	42
	87	42
	42	75
	27	87
	98	98
	114	109
	75	114

(These examples and much of the text was contributed by Robert Fontaine with help from ASC Ehrenberg [16].)

Use the table layout effectively to help the viewer --
place numbers for comparison close together

Year	Both Sexes	Male	Female
1973	600	500	99
1970	670	580	87
1968	550	460	89
1966	330	260	71

Draw columns and rows close together

Year	Both Sexes	Male	Female
1973	600	500	99
1970	670	580	87
1968	550	460	89
1966	330	260	71

Move and minimize intervening numbers

Year	Rate per 1000 (SE)						
	Male		Female		All	
1993	83	(2.3)	78	(2.2)	80	(1.9)
1994	62	(2.5)	66	(2.7)	63	(1.8)
1995	58	(2.1)	54	(2.0)	56	(1.7)
1996	55	(2.0)	45	(2.0)	51	(1.7)

Remove intervening numbers entirely
if consequence minimal

Year	Rate per 1000[a]		
	M	F	All
1993	83	78	80
1994	62	66	63
1995	58	54	56
1996	55	45	51

a. Standard errors for all rates less than 5% of rate.

Organize data by magnitude

Exposure	1000 Cases	Rate	Rate Ratio	p
A	11	2.9	1.3	> 0.10
B	6	9.9	4.3	< 0.001
C	34	5.4	2.3	> 0.1
None	27	2.3	1.0	Ref*

a = p-value
b = reference exposure category

Organize data by magnitude

Exposure	1000 Cases	Rate	Rate Ratio	p[a]
B	6	9.9	4.3	< 0.01
C	34	5.4	2.3	< 0.05
A	11	2.9	1.3	> 0.001
None	27	2.3	1.0	Ref[b]

a. = p-value
b. = reference exposure category

7.11   Using Less Informative Denominators in a Table

Multicolumn tables allow readers to compare characteristics among different subgroups. Authors commonly include percentages to assist data interpretation. Sometimes, authors erroneously report percentages using less informative row totals as the denominator rather than the more informative column denominator.

Using a row total denominator prevents an intuitive comparison of the columns, thereby undermining a primary advantage of presenting data in tables.

Consider the two tables below that describe study subjects some of whom were enrolled near battery recycling sites and others who were enrolled near turmeric processing sites. Some of the study subjects were caregivers, and some were workers.

In the erroneous table at the top, row totals are used to calculate proportions. Thus, among the 188 illiterate study subjects, 74% of them were caregivers who were enrolled at the battery recycling site. By comparison, only 5% were caregivers who were enrolled at the turmeric processing site. This comparison is not particularly informative. It reflects the peculiarity of study subject enrollment. Specifically, that more study subjects were enrolled from battery recycling rather than from turmeric processing. If the study team had spent a few more days at turmeric processing sites, these numbers would be quite different. The proportions do not reflect underlying characteristics of the different groups. The proportion in the total column is particularly uninformative.

The proportions in the alternative table are more informative. They illustrate, for example, that 31% of caregivers at the battery recycling site were illiterate in contrast to 16% in the turmeric processing site and 100% of workers. It suggests that these groups are different.

Examples of the error:

× **Table.** Demographic and socio-economic information of the respondents.

Characteristics	Caregivers			
	Battery recycling site (n=444)	Turmeric processing site (n=57)	Workers (n=40)	Total (N=541)
Age				
Mean	31.4	32.1	37.6	31.9
Educational status				
Illiterate	139 (74%)	9 (5%)	40 (21%)	188 (100%)
Monthly household income				
Mean ± SD	16739	18139	15756	16808
Occupation				
Dependent	422 (89%)	55 (11%)	0 (0%)	477 (100%)

Alternative, better option:

✓ **Table.** Demographic and socio-economic information of the respondents.

Characteristics	Caregivers			
	Battery recycling site (n=444)	Turmeric processing site (n=57)	Workers (n=40)	Total (N=541)
Age				
Mean	31.4	32.1	37.6	31.9
Educational status				
Illiterate	139 (31%)	9 (16%)	40 (100%)	188 (35%)
Monthly household income				
Mean ± SD	16739	18139	15756	16808
Occupation				
Dependent	422 (95%)	55 (97%)	0 (0%)	477 (88%)

7.12   Comparing to a Varying Baseline

We often analyze data where observations are grouped into multiple levels of exposure. In the example below, we have categorized observed handwashing behavior into mutually exclusive categories:

Handwashing after defecation	Group A		Group B		Odds ratio	
					varying	reference
	Number	%	Number	%	baseline	group
No handwashing	75	12%	150	19%	0.6	--
Washed one hand with water alone	150	23%	150	19%	1.3	2.0
Washed both hands with water alone	125	19%	150	19%	1.0	1.7
Washed one hand with soap	150	23%	100	15%	2.1	3.0
Washed both hands with soap	150	23%	200	25%	0.9	1.5
Total	650		750			

The common error is to compare the prevalence of each level of the variable in group A to the prevalence at the same level of the variable in group B. Thus, if we compare the prevalence of washing both hands with water alone, the prevalence is the same (19%) in group A and group B, so we could say that people in group A and B are equally likely to wash both hands with water alone, which is equivalent to an odds ratio of 1.0. The problem with this comparison is that the people who are not washing both hands with water alone are quite a heterogeneous group. Some of them are practicing less intense handwashing (not washing their hands at all or only washing one hand), and others are practicing more intense handwashing. Indeed, even if we have an elevated odds ratio with such a comparison, it is difficult to interpret because we don't know if this elevation results from a difference in more intense or less intense handwashing.

The standard approach to resolve this dilemma is to arrange the exposure level into a mutually exclusive hierarchy. Set the lowest level of exposure as the reference group, and then consider the 2 × 2 table comparing each level of exposure to this reference group. Using this approach illustrated in the final column, we can conclude that compared with group B, group A is more likely to wash either one or both hands with water rather than not washing at all.

7.13   P-Value in a Baseline Table of a Randomized Controlled Trial

In a randomized controlled trial, the intervention is assigned randomly. Therefore, any difference between groups is due to random assignment. A p-value tests whether or not an observed difference is larger than would be expected by chance. It is an irrelevant test in a randomized controlled trial.

If reviewers asked that such a comparison be added to your baseline table, cite the classic article: Altman D. Comparability of randomised groups. *The Statistician* (1985) 34, pp. 125–136. If you believe your reviewer has a sense of humor, you may want to directly quote from Altman, " . . . Performing a significance test to compare baseline variables is to assess the probability of something having occurred by chance when we know that it did occur by chance. Such a procedure is clearly absurd."

It remains important to assess whether there are meaningful differences between the intervention and control group. If there is imbalance, this suggests that randomization failed to create balanced group. If the baseline characteristics that differ between groups are also associated with the study outcome, then an adjusted analysis will need to be included. The assessment of baseline differences, however, is not based on evaluating a p-value but rather on a judgment of whether the differences in characteristics between groups is large enough that they could plausibly affect the outcome.

Examples of the error:

✗ Table 1: Student household characteristics at baseline (N=1,560)

Description	Intervention (N=688) n (%)	Control (N=872) n (%)	*p* value
Source of household income			
Formal employment/service	405 (59)	479 (55)	0.12
Self-employment	27 (4)	43 (5)	0.34
Casual/contract job	57 (8)	95 (11)	0.08
Day labor	102 (15)	93 (11)	0.01
Rikshaw/van puller	46 (7)	99 (11)	0.002
Driving motor vehicles	51 (7)	63 (7)	0.89
Household size (member): Mean (Std. Dev.)	5.0 (1.6)	4.9 (1.5)	0.32

Alternative, better option:

✓ Table 1: Student household characteristics at baseline (N=1,560)

Description	Intervention (N=688) n (%)	Control (N=872) n (%)
Source of household income		
Formal employment/service	405 (59)	479 (55)
Self-employment	27 (4)	43 (5)
Casual/contract job	57 (8)	95 (11)
Day labor	102 (15)	93 (11)
Rikshaw/van puller	46 (7)	99 (11)
Driving motor vehicles	51 (7)	63 (7)
Household size (member): Mean (Std. Dev.)	5.0 (1.6)	4.9 (1.5)

7.14 Using Nonstandard Footnote Symbols in Tables

Footnotes contribute important explanations to data presented in tables. They are useful to clarify an analytic approach, groups being compared, statistical significance, and other explanatory information. Historically, the sequence of footnotes was:

*, †, ‡, §, ||, ¶, **, ††, ‡‡, §§, ||||, ¶¶, etc.

You can find these symbols using the insert symbol feature of Microsoft Word. Note that these symbols should be in superscript.

More recently, some journals have suggested different symbols (most commonly a, b, c, d...). Check with your target journal's instructions to authors to ensure that your notation is consistent with their preference.

7.15   Using the Wrong Symbol to Designate Degree

Wrong example: 4 0C or 4 oC
    To use the degree symbol, select the insert symbol feature of Word, select a circle (i.e., not the letter "o" or the number zero), and then make the circle superscript.
    Correct example: 4 °C
    Recent versions of MS Word include a degree symbol. Go to Insert and then Symbol to find the figure.

7.16   Numbering Figures or Tables out of Sequence

Readers expect and journals require tables and figures to be numbered in the order that they are referred to in the narrative text of the paper (i.e., Table 1, Table 2, Table 3, Figure 1, Figure 2, Figure 3). In addition, each table and figure should be cited in the narrative text (otherwise, readers and editors will assume it is not important and can be dropped).
    The most common form of this error is when authors mention an element of complicated data analysis in the methods section and refer to a later table or figure in the manuscript. Usually, the best approach in this situation is to describe the statistical method without pointing to the results table or figure. The problem with citing the advanced table or figure as Table 1 or Figure 1 is that it will confuse readers to have this more complicated analysis presented before the more basic results that build toward the more complicated analysis.
    The other common form of this error is renumbering the tables or figures but not updating these numbers in the narrative text.

7.17   Maps with Irrelevant Details

When a map is included in the manuscript, its role is to communicate specific geographical information, for example, the location of the study, spatial relationships among cases, or the spatial distribution of exposures. Inserting a map constructed by someone else that is filled with details that are irrelevant to the communication role for the map, for example, district divisions, rivers, or railroad lines, distracts readers from the message. Draw your own map or begin with a generic map and add the elements that are essential to the message.

Example of the error

Alternative, better option

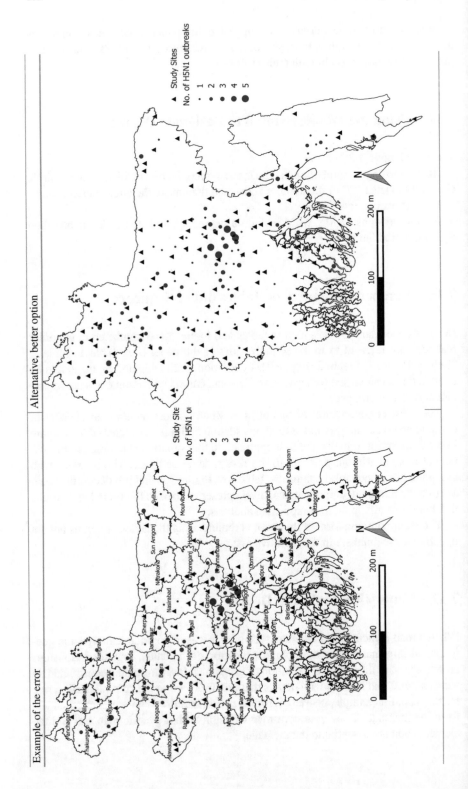

Open Access This chapter is licensed under the terms of the Creative Commons Attribution 4.0 International License (http://creativecommons.org/licenses/by/4.0/), which permits use, sharing, adaptation, distribution and reproduction in any medium or format, as long as you give appropriate credit to the original author(s) and the source, provide a link to the Creative Commons license and indicate if changes were made.

The images or other third party material in this chapter are included in the chapter's Creative Commons license, unless indicated otherwise in a credit line to the material. If material is not included in the chapter's Creative Commons license and your intended use is not permitted by statutory regulation or exceeds the permitted use, you will need to obtain permission directly from the copyright holder.

Chapter 8
Approaching Publication

8.1 Failure to Respond to Reviewers' Comments

The first author has the right to decide what will ultimately be included in the manuscript and how it will be framed. Nevertheless, a first author should respond to every issue raised by a reviewer or co-author. It is acceptable to reject the offered advice. In a scientific environment, co-authors and other reviewers fully expect that some of their advice will be rejected. Indeed, it is important to reject inappropriate or unsound advice. However, if you choose to reject the advice of a reviewer or a co-author, you need to defend that decision when you submit the next draft.

To address every point raised by a reviewer, either change the manuscript accordingly, or explain in a separate note the issues you chose not to change and defend why you chose not to change them. If you simply ignore the advice, you will receive the same comments from the co-author/reviewer again. The paper will not develop further. Both the reviewer and author will feel that their time is being wasted. Often, this situation reflects a communication problem. The reviewer does not understand something that is very clear to the author. Reviewer comments can be an important clue that the author should work to make the narrative more understandable. The key is to respond to every issue raised by a reviewer. Be prepared to continue to revise even after submission to a journal.

8.2 Incomplete Response to External Reviews

When responding to comments, the goal is not to provide a minimalist justification why you wrote what you wrote. Instead, the task is to demonstrate to co-authors, editors, and reviewers that you fully understand the critique and the implication of the critique for your paper. If the reviewer raises a meaningful issue, you need to

© The Author(s) 2022
S. Luby, D. L. Southern, *The Pathway to Publishing: A Guide to Quantitative Writing in the Health Sciences*, https://doi.org/10.1007/978-3-030-98175-4_8

respond to that critique and revise the manuscript so that other readers do not face similar questions and confusion.

Indeed, this is one of the great benefits of having your work undergo peer review. We should not lament that "the reviewer did not understand our work" or that the reviewer did not see that the current text already addressed their question. If the reviewer did not understand, we should take this as a signal that our message was not written clearly enough to be readily understood and consider what changes we can make to the paper so that future readers will not suffer the same misunderstanding.

It is completely acceptable, indeed expected, to disagree with some points made by a reviewer or co-author, but such disagreement must be framed within the context of a full understanding of their critique. For a manuscript that is resubmitted to a journal, the editor will review the responses carefully and may ask the reviewer(s) to look again at the manuscript and your responses.

8.2.1 Not Including Text of the Manuscript Changes in Response to External Reviewers

In response to external reviews, the author drafts a response document (Sect. 1.3.2). The editor and reviewers should be able to understand this document by reading it beginning to end, without having to simultaneously check the revised manuscript. The response to reviewer document should clarify the specific changes you made in the manuscript as a response to each comment. The manuscript revisions should be included in the response document clearly noted in quotation marks or through other format signaling. These direct quotations from the revised manuscript may be as short as a clarifying restatement of a phrase or a sentence or as long as one or more paragraphs.

If you change the manuscript, but don't make it clear in the response document that you made these changes, then the editor has to go point by point and try to figure out what you changed and what you did not change. This is a painstaking, frustrating, and annoying task. If you want your manuscript to be accepted, avoid annoying the editor. Demonstrate to the editor that you have thoroughly considered and responded to each of these issues. Make it easy for the editor to accept your work.

8.3 Invalid Authorship Line

Inclusion on an author line is an important indicator of one's contribution to scientific work and an important professional credential. The authorship line can sometimes be controversial, so it is important to understand who should be included and who should not. All writers should read the "Recommendations for the Conduct,

Reporting, Editing, and Publication of Scholarly Work in Medical Journals," a document developed by the International Committee of Medical Journal Editors (ICMJE) available at www.icmje.org. Essentially, authorship credit should be based on four criteria with authors meeting each criteria:

- Substantial contributions to the conception or design of the work or the acquisition, analysis, or interpretation of data for the work
- Drafting the work or revising it critically for important intellectual content
- Final approval of the version to be published
- Agreement to be accountable for all aspects of the work and ensuring that questions related to the accuracy or integrity of any part of the work are appropriately investigated and resolved

If you follow these guidelines, your choices can be defended in any academic setting. Clarify in your own mind who clearly fulfills the criteria for authorship. Have a separate discussion with your supervisor if you believe that any other person should be included, for example, a government colleague who is critical to the government acting on the manuscript recommendations or an institutional collaborator who is essential to support ongoing scientific collaboration. Know your institutional or program criteria.

Guidance on developing an author line is provided in Sect. 1.2.4, and a tool, the authorship ranking scorecard, for assigning authorship is included in Appendix 8.

This tool helps to clarify who should be included as an author on a paper, and the ordinal ranking of the authors. We recommend that you use this authorship scorecard to share your suggestions for authorship with your primary reviewer when you develop your framing document.

8.4 Retaining Comments in Subsequent Drafts

Many co-authors make comments on draft manuscripts using the comment feature of word processors. These can provide useful input to the author. Often, the authors are tempted to respond to comments by continuing the conversation within a series of comment bubbles. The result is the next draft includes two conversations. First is the narrative text. Second is a side conversation among co-authors. Complex drafts that include a lot of historical commentary from multiple reviewers are burdensome and distracting to review.

The goal in drafting a scientific manuscript is a narrative text that is clear and stands on its own. Readers of the published manuscript will not have access to all of the side commentary. The task of a scientific author is to write clearly and strive to address the primary concerns of most readers. Responding in comment form risks Error 8.2.

Retaining a couple of comments that are addressing central issues where there is some appropriate conversation can be helpful, but these should be minimized so that the focus remains on creating a clear text that stands on its own.

If there are a number of comments from co-authors that would benefit from explaining why you did not take certain suggestions (Error 8.1), this is often better communicated by a separate response document. Each co-author can see that their issues were considered, but the main document remains self-explanatory. Alternatively, you can circulate a clean and marked version. The marked version can have detailed responses to comments and show track changes, but the clean document is the working document that presents the draft close to how a new reader would see it.

Example of the Error

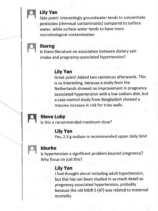

Not only does the salinity affect water taste—resulting in many people abandoning these tube wells for surface water sources like ponds or rivers which are more likely to have microbiological contamination (9,10)—it is also correlated with pregnancy-associated hypertension (5,11). Pregnancy-associated hypertension encompasses a disease spectrum from simple hypertension to eclampsia with seizures, and accounts for 20% of maternal mortality in Bangladesh (12,13). The link between dietary salt intake and traditional hypertension is well known, and in southwest Bangladesh average sodium intake from tube well water jumps from 0.6-1.2 g/day in the rainy season to 5-16 g/day in the dry season, which is more than double the recommended maximum daily dose (11,14). Furthermore, women whose primary drinking source is a tube well have a 8.15 OR of gestational hypertension or (pre)eclampsia compared to women who use rainwater (15). While current studies examining dietary salt intake and pregnancy-associated hypertension show no improvement with low sodium diets, they do not examine possible risks of very high sodium intake (16). Reducing the salinity of underground aquifers may reduce the prevalence of pregnancy associated hypertension in coastal regions.

Alternative, Better Option

Not only does the salinity affect water taste—resulting in many people abandoning these tube wells for surface water sources like ponds or rivers which are more likely to have microbiological contamination (9,10)—it is also correlated with pregnancy-associated hypertension (5,11). Pregnancy-associated hypertension encompasses a disease spectrum from simple hypertension to eclampsia with seizures, and accounts for 20% of maternal mortality in Bangladesh (12,13). The link between dietary salt intake and traditional hypertension is well known, and in southwest Bangladesh average sodium intake from tube well water jumps from 0.6-1.2 g/day in the rainy season to 5-16 g/day in the dry season, which is more than double the recommended maximum daily dose (11,14). Furthermore, women whose primary drinking source is a tube well have a 8.15 OR of gestational hypertension or (pre)eclampsia compared to women who use rainwater (15). While current studies examining dietary salt intake and pregnancy-associated hypertension show no improvement with low sodium diets, they do not examine possible risks of very high sodium intake (16). Reducing the salinity of underground aquifers may reduce the prevalence of pregnancy associated hypertension in coastal regions.

8.5   Choosing an Inappropriate Journal

It is rarely obvious which journal is best for your article. Many early career scientists request their senior author to recommend the target journal. This approach undercuts the opportunity to learn how to choose a journal. Instead, early career scientists should consider candidate journals and then propose and defend a prioritized list of journals to their senior author. By considering feedback from their senior author and ultimately their own experience in attempting to publish in various journals, authors can develop and hone their judgment regarding optimal journal choice.

Choosing a journal depends on whom is the best audience for your research question. Explore some journals by reviewing previous issues. Have they published similar studies? Look at the references from an up-to-date manuscript you have found during your literature search. Do you see any journals where this type of paper has been published? Look more closely at journals that have either published work on the topic engaged by your manuscript or published articles using similar methods as your manuscript on analogous topics.

Another consideration is the journal's impact factor. The impact factor is a measure of the frequency that the "average article" published in a given scholarly journal has been cited in a particular year or period. This metric reflects the importance of communication in scientific work. As science is a social activity, articles that are noted and cited by other researchers are influencing the field. This factor is often used to measure or describe the importance of a particular journal to its field. The Institute for Scientific Information ranks, evaluates, and compares journals within subject categories and annually publishes the results in Journal Citation Reports.

The formula to determine impact factor 2020 for a journal would be calculated as follows:

A = the number of times articles published in 2018–19 were cited in indexed journals during 2020

B = the number of articles, reviews, proceedings, or notes published in 2018–19

Impact factor 2020 = A/B

Impact factors can have a controversial influence on the way published scientific research is perceived and evaluated. Criticism of using impact factors as a measure of journal quality include:

- Journal impact factors depend on the research field: High impact factors are more likely in journals covering large areas of basic research and less likely in more subject-specific journals.
- Although Journal Citation Reports include some non-English journals, the index is heavily skewed toward English-language journals, leaving out important international sources.
- Researchers may be more likely to pursue fashionable topics that have a higher likelihood of being published in a high-impact journal than to follow important avenues that may not be as popular.
- Review articles are often highly cited, but they make a different contribution than highly cited original work.

Because there are so many journals today, and because most scholars look for articles using electronic search engines, the impact factor of the journal may be less important now than it was a generation ago. Many very highly cited articles are published in journals that do not have a particularly high average impact factor. You want to select a journal whose editors will be interested in your work and who are able to identify good peer reviewers. Often, a specialty journal with a somewhat lower impact factor is the best place to reach readers interested in your topic and where journal editors can find high-quality reviewers.

Good reviewers identify important issues for further development in your manuscript. Good reviewers improve your manuscript. Better manuscripts have more influence. If you have results that you and your supervisor believe represent broad scientific interest, it is reasonable to submit it to a more competitive high-impact journal. Recognize, however, that these high-impact journals, for example, the *Lancet, Science,* or *Nature,* reject >90% of submitted manuscripts. Each manuscript submission takes time, time that could be deployed in writing your next manuscript.

Consider whether reaching for a high-impact journal for a special manuscript is a good investment of time. Publishing in a high-impact journal could help draw attention to your findings. It might send a useful signal to potential employers about the quality of your scientific work. On the other hand, using your manuscript writing time to prepare your next manuscript can also add to both your scientific contribution and your reputation. Submitting to journals where the type of work that you are submitting is commonly published can save valuable time. For help with finding appropriate journals, explore the website JANE (Appendix 10).

8.6 Not Following a Specific Journal's Details of Style

All journals periodically publish their style rules in a hard copy edition, or these style rules are always available on the journals' website under "Instructions for Authors" or "Requirements for Manuscripts." Go online and read the individual journal's instructions and follow them closely before you submit your manuscript.

8.7 Not Using an Appropriate Reporting Guideline

After your manuscript is published, it will be read, critically appraised, and hopefully will contribute to systematic reviews, inform specific public health guidelines, and influence overall public health practice. Before you submit your paper to a journal, you should consider if you have provided enough details so that the work can be used for these additional purposes.

A number of guidelines have been developed to help to prevent inadequate reporting of research activities. The Strengthening the Reporting of Observational Studies in Epidemiology (**STROBE**) statement is for observational studies, **CONSORT** is for randomized controlled trials, **PRISMA** for systematic reviews with or without meta-analysis or other statistical synthesis methods, and **STARD** for studies of diagnostic accuracy. A comprehensive list of the available reporting guidelines appropriate for a wide variety of different study types is available at the Enhancing the QUAlity and Transparency Of health Research (EQUATOR) Network library for health research reporting guidelines at https://www.equator-network.org/reporting-guidelines/.

The International Committee of Medical Journal Editors (www.icmje.org) encourages journals to ask authors to follow these guidelines because they help authors describe the study in enough detail for it to be evaluated by editors, reviewers, readers, and other researchers. Some peer-reviewed journals require authors to follow a pertinent guideline.

Researchers should use these guidelines to review their paper to make sure all information is included.

8.8 Exceeding the Journal Word Limit

Exceeding your target journal's word limit for manuscript length, especially for an initial submission, increases the risk that the editor will reject the paper without sending it for external review. The most common form of this error is an author circulating a draft manuscript that is over the journal word limit and then asking co-authors to edit the draft for them.

It is an art to write succinctly, an art that is valuable to cultivate because readers' attention is a scarce resource, and holding readers' attention with your scientific writing is essential for your ideas to influence global scientific discourse.

An initial draft circulated to co-authors may be a little long, but do not circulate a late-stage draft of the manuscript where either the abstract or the body of the manuscript exceeds the specifications of the target journal.

When your manuscript is less than 15–20% over limit, and you've had one or more rounds of input from co-authors, dedicate several hours to reviewing every single sentence and asking yourself, "How can I communicate these ideas clearly with fewer words?" Smile every time you reduce a couple of words, and cheer when you realize you can drop a whole sentence by reorganizing your arguments and dropping some repetition. If you specifically focus on succinct language, you can often markedly reduce word count without eliminating ideas. Focusing on writing succinctly increases the clarity of your scientific reasoning. This laborious task is a first author responsibility.

A version of this error is circulating a draft manuscript with an abstract that is much longer than permitted by your target journal. It is a poor use of your co-author's time to review a draft abstract that is so underdeveloped that you have not addressed the central task of an abstract, which is succinctly summarizing the manuscript within the space and format restrictions of the target journal. We recommend that co-authors refuse to review any abstract that is more than 10% over the word limit. Instead, first authors should exert the effort so that the abstract is a genuine draft abstract formatted for the target journal. An abstract of the appropriate length and format respects co-authors' time and encourages focused and useful suggestions.

8.9   Asking Your Senior Author to Recommend Reviewers

Many journals request that authors recommend reviewers at the time of manuscript submission. This assists editors because authors are in a good position to identify people who are expert in the area of their submitted work. If an early career author asks a senior author for a list of potential reviewers, then he/she undermines the opportunity to learn how to select reviewers.

A good reviewer is someone who would be interested in your work and has published work that is closely enough related that he or she would have an informed opinion. A good place to begin is considering the authors of the references cited within your manuscript. Also conduct some brief literature searches, and review abstracts to identify other potential candidates. When considering subject matter to search, consider not only the central subject of your manuscript but also related subjects or authors who have reported work using a similar method.

More senior scientists will have more requests for reviews and so will likely decline to review a larger proportion of review requests. Scientists who have very recently published in a related subject area may be particularly interested in providing a review.

Draw up a list of reviewers, provide a reason for selecting each reviewer, and then ask for input from your senior author. This way, you will both generate a reasonable list of reviewers and have gained experience to help you select reviewers for future articles.

8.10   Responding to Journal Reviewers Using the First Person Singular

In group-authored papers, the manuscript is the product of the work of the group. All authors agree to publically defend what is written. Similarly, the response to reviewers is not only what the author who drafted the response is saying; it is a statement from all authors. Once you have responded to external reviews, you should provide all co-authors a 1-week opportunity to review those comments and make any suggestions. (Early career authors should first have their senior author review the response to reviewers before circulating to all authors.) Because the responses to reviewers reflect the combined responses of all authors, the first person singular "I" should not be used in the response document.

Examples of the error		Alternative, better options	
✗	I have revised the related text to provide the details of the selection process of the informants.	✓	We have revised the related text to provide the details of the selection process of the informants.
✗	I have tried my best to address all of your major and minor comments.	✓	We have addressed each of the comments.

8.11 Missing Acknowledgment Section

Many research organizations and academic institutions have a specific policy, template, and language for acknowledging the financial or material assistance from the agency or government that funded your research. Check your institution's policy. Confirm the donor's grant number by reviewing the contract. Government donors often require a statement that the conclusions of the article are the authors' own and should not be construed as official government policy. Clarify from the donor the specific language that they prefer.

People who contributed to the study, but do not fulfill the criteria for co-authorship, should be listed in the acknowledgment section. These may include:

- Community members of the study site
- Data collectors
- Laboratory support
- Administrative support
- Statistical assistance
- Writing assistance

Look at examples of the acknowledgment section from the journal you are planning to submit to. The wording is usually professional in tone. Journals commonly require that anyone listed by name in the acknowledgment section must agree to have their name listed. If you want to acknowledge a person by name, send an email requesting permission to list his/her contribution in the acknowledgments section. If he/she responds affirmatively, simply save the email in case a question is raised by the journal editor.

8.12 Reusing an Email Thread when Circulating a Revised Manuscript

Many email programs organize emails in "threads." As long as people keep responding to the email, the email program will group these emails together. When an author sends a revised version of a manuscript using the thread from their previous draft, they risk generating confusion. A long thread containing multiple drafts requires your co-authors to sort through the thread and try to figure out which is the most recent draft. It can be confusing because co-authors provide feedback on different drafts. This wastes co-authors time. In the worst case, co-authors dedicate substantial time to reviewing an outdated draft. The solution is straightforward. Each draft should be circulated with a new email thread. Use the subject line to specify draft-specific information. You can generate the addressees by copying and pasting from the email from the prior draft.

8.13 Requesting an Unprofessionally Short Turnaround Time

Asking others to be a co-author is requesting that they assume a substantial responsibility. By affiliating their name with the article, co-authors are accepting accountability for the work. They are publically connecting their reputation to the quality and the veracity of the scientific work, its analysis, and its interpretation. Assuming this responsibility requires careful review of the draft manuscript and ensuring that important issues are resolved prior to submission.

Co-authors are busy. Knowledge workers characteristically have more demands on their time than they have time in a day. When you request that co-authors give time to your article, you should be sensitive to how much of a request this is and so provide a reasonable time for co-authors to respond (Sect. 1.2.5).

In the absence of exceptional extenuating circumstances, asking for a review within a few days communicates a lack of professionalism and a lack of respect to co-authors. It is not a recipe for productive long-term collaboration.

Examples of the error		Alternative, better options	
✗	Attached is the final version of our paper. Please send me your consent to be a co-author by tomorrow so we can proceed with journal submission.	✓	Attached is the most recent version of our paper. I have attempted to address all of the concerns raised by co-authors. I am anxious to proceed with submission. Please look over the draft, and if you concur, please send a statement that you agree to be listed as a co-author and agree with its submission for publication. Of course, any additional suggestions to improve the paper, would be welcome. Please respond by (give specific date; 2 weeks after email is sent).

8.14 Sending Blank Forms for Co-authors to Complete

Journals often require signed forms from co-authors reflecting their contribution to the manuscript, their willingness to be included as a co-author, and declarations of potential conflicts of interest. These forms typically require the name of the manuscript and other details that are the same for all co-authors, but also some information specific for each co-author. Both as a courtesy to your colleagues, as well as to boost team efficiency, before circulating these forms the first author should complete as much of the form as possible so that, for example, each co-author doesn't need to go back through their files and find out what the exact title of the manuscript is.

8.15 Not Providing Co-authors a Copy of the Submitted Manuscript

Co-authored manuscripts reflect the collective work of the whole team of authors. When submitting a manuscript to a journal, most journal websites generate a PDF version of what was actually submitted or allow the submitting author to generate such a document. A copy of this document should be provided to all co-authors so that each has the most up-to-date version of the group's collective work. This way, if questions arise about the article or the analysis prior to publication, co-authors have access to the best collective understanding.

8.16 Not Keeping Co-authors Informed of Discussion with Journal Editors

Co-authored manuscripts reflect the collective work of all the authors. When editors and reviewers raise concerns, this discussion is relevant to the whole co-author team. The best practice is to circulate comments as soon as they are received so that all co-authors can consider them. Next, the first author should respond to each of the critiques and make appropriate changes in the manuscript. Often, there are several iterations of responses to revisions between the first author and the senior author. Once the senior author is satisfied, then the first author should send around the responses and manuscript changes to all co-authors for their input. It is best to give co-authors 1 week to review this. Journals often set deadlines for when responses and revisions need to be returned, so it is best to begin working on these revisions promptly to allow the opportunity for all co-authors to weigh in and improve the collective responses and so the final manuscript.

The exception to this approach is when the editor has asked for only minor changes in style or correction of a couple minor errors. Then it is more efficient to simply respond to the journal and send a copy to all co-authors of the responses and the revised submission.

8.17 Emailing Draft Manuscripts with Figures That Are Not Compressed

Figures, especially high-resolution photographs, require a large amount of computer memory. Frequently, a single photograph takes more than five times as much space as all of the text and all of the references in a document. For reviewers, most of this is wasted space. The figure is at a much higher level of resolution than would ever be discernible in publication or is even discernible on the reviewer's computer screens. These large files increase transit times, clog up email, and consume hard drive space. It is inconsiderate to send these unnecessarily massive files to co-authors for review. Remember, you are asking busy reviewers to give time to provide feedback on your manuscript. Making this as easy as possible generates goodwill from these key stakeholders.

If you use Microsoft Word, you can compress these pictures through the following:

1. Click on the picture.
2. Navigate on the format tab, and click on the Compress Picture icon.
3. This dialog box will appear:

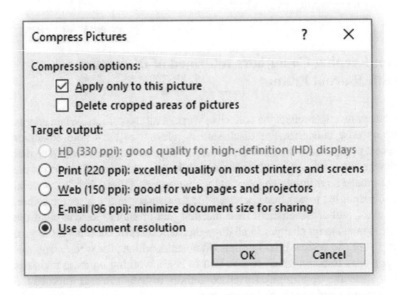

4. Uncheck "Apply only to this picture."
5. Check "Web" or "Email."
6. Click on OK.

If you use a different word processor, look on the internet for instructions on how to compress pictures/figures.

Sometimes, statistical analysis software will generate statistically dense outputs in PDF format. These can be dozens or hundreds of megabytes large and take minutes to load. Again, the resolution is beyond what a computer screen can display and what the human eye can discern. A simple solution for Windows users is to use the snipping tool to take an image of the output and paste this into the PDF. Other operating systems have a similar function. This will show the identical detail but not hog resources.

8.18   Not Including Readability Statistics

Scientific articles are more likely to be cited and more likely to influence the world if they are easily understood. A simple way to improve the readability of your manuscript is to use tools that track readability so that you can adjust your prose to make it more understandable. Many word processing software programs include a readability assessment tool that can quickly analyze your draft. Alternatively, several websites offer easy-to-use readability tools. If you open your favorite search engine and enter the phrase "online readability checker," you can choose from several options.

The most common metrics to consider include the following:

1. Average words per sentence should be <25. Strive to be concise.
2. Readability:

    (a) Flesch Reading Ease on a scale of 1–100. A higher number means that the manuscript is easier to read. Strive for >50.
    (a) Flesch-Kincaid Grade level is based on US schools with 19.7 being a professional or PhD level. A lower number means that it is easier to read. Target a grade level of 16–18.

Open Access   This chapter is licensed under the terms of the Creative Commons Attribution 4.0 International License (http://creativecommons.org/licenses/by/4.0/), which permits use, sharing, adaptation, distribution and reproduction in any medium or format, as long as you give appropriate credit to the original author(s) and the source, provide a link to the Creative Commons license and indicate if changes were made.

The images or other third party material in this chapter are included in the chapter's Creative Commons license, unless indicated otherwise in a credit line to the material. If material is not included in the chapter's Creative Commons license and your intended use is not permitted by statutory regulation or exceeds the permitted use, you will need to obtain permission directly from the copyright holder.

Chapter 9
Slide and Poster Presentations

9.1 Bullets on the Wall

Bullets on the wall are slides that present a detailed outline of the talk as bullet points that are projected on the screen/poster board. In the days before slides and screen protectors, speakers commonly used an outline as a prompt to help remember the key points of their talk. A written outline of the ideas that you want to cover in a talk remains a useful aid to a complete and coherent presentation, especially if you are speaking without slides. However, projecting a detailed outline of your talk on the wall, and then talking through the points bullet by bullet, or even worse, reading them directly to the audience, is a misuse of the verbal presentation format and a huge turnoff to the audience.

Do you like attending oral presentations where bullets are projected on the wall and the speaker reads them to you? When a Fortune 500 company has a new product to advertise, do they use a bulleted list to communicate its attributes to potential customers? Of course not. We are drawn to engaging speakers and engaging presentations. One of the roles of a scientist is to communicate her/his findings and ideas so that a broader audience considers them, so it affects the audience's understanding and impacts serious discussions.

A verbal presentation is an opportunity to leverage a range of your interpersonal skills to communicate your ideas with your audience. For centuries, people have made compelling oral presentations without visual aids. The slides that support an oral presentation should be constructed to reinforce your communication objectives, so it helps the audience understand the ideas you are presenting. Bullets after bullets after bullets bore an audience. This is a recipe for losing the audience's attention and failing to meet your communication objectives (Figs. 9.1.1 and 9.1.2).

© The Author(s) 2022
S. Luby, D. L. Southern, *The Pathway to Publishing: A Guide to Quantitative Writing in the Health Sciences*, https://doi.org/10.1007/978-3-030-98175-4_9

Background

- Respiratory viruses can cause pandemics and epidemics
- Emergence of Severe Respiratory Distress Syndrome (SARS) led WHO to revise, adopt and implement the IHR (2005) to detect emerging pathogens
- Strong surveillance systems are the cornerstone of pandemic preparedness and response
- Early detection of unusual clusters in human to human transmission as the most important function of surveillance
- Individual disease cluster investigations may not be fruitful unless the causal mechanism is single and the relative risk is high
- Investigation of clustering of a given disease detects space-time aggregation of cases which is caused by environmental agents

Background cont'd

- Proactive identification systems can enable public health officials to identify problems earlier

- Bangladesh, a densely populated country with widespread influenza H5N1 outbreaks in poultry is a particularly high risk for emergence of new strains with pandemic potential

- In 2007, ICDDRB set up national hospital-based influenza surveillance in collaboration with the Government of Bangladesh Institute of Epidemiology Disease Control and Research

- In 2009, ICDDRB embedded cluster investigations into the surveillance system to identify new strains and the viral etiology of clusters of severe respiratory infections

Fig. 9.1.1 Opening slides for an influenza surveillance talk with too many bullets

1918-1919 Influenza Pandemic

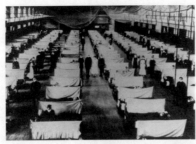

30 – 100 million deaths globally in 9 months
- 2.5% of infected persons died
- >25 times the typical rate for influenza

Photo : US Public Health Service

Fig. 9.1.2 An alternative opening slide for an influenza surveillance talk that communicates to the audience why this is a compelling issue

9.2   Using Sentences for Bullet Points

Bullet points should be terse summaries that help the audience follow your key points. They should not be full sentences or paragraphs that you read. Full sentences and paragraphs are appropriate for scientific writing, but it is mind-numbingly boring to have full sentence after full sentence projected with the speaker reading the sentences to the audience. The average audience member can read such sentences three to five times faster than the presenter can speak them, so this is not an efficient method to communicate. It is a misuse of a verbal presentation opportunity.

Posters are meant to be read, and so somewhat longer lines of text can be used than in a verbal presentation, but ideas that break down into sections should still be presented as brief bullet points so people can quickly grasp the structure of the ideas (Figs. 9.2.1, 9.2.2, 9.2.3, and 9.2.4).

Definition and data analysis

- We defined a toilet is clean if there was an "absence of feces, liquids or dirt within the squatting area and pan of the toilet"

- To identify the factors associated with toilet cleanliness we estimated the prevalence ratio (PR) using generalized estimating equations to account for clustering

Fig. 9.2.1 Sentences making minimal use of visual organization of ideas

Definition and data analysis

Clean toilet:
- absence of
  - Feces
  - Liquids
  - Dirt
- within
  - Squatting area
  - Pan

To identify the factors associated with toilet cleanliness
- prevalence ratios
- generalized estimating equations to account for clustering

Fig. 9.2.2 Ideas organized as bullets. This would also accommodate a nice picture of a clean toilet which would further enhance communication

Fig. 9.2.3 Paragraph-like
bullet from a draft poster

• In courtyard meetings, participants received
  messages to wash hands with soap after
  defecation, after cleaning a child's anus and
  before preparing food. Handwashing before
  child feeding was not included in the
  promotional messages

Fig. 9.2.4 Information
recast as quick-to-read
organized bullets

• In courtyard meetings, participants received
  messages to wash hands with soap:
    −after defecation
    −after cleaning a child's anus
    −before preparing food.

• Handwashing before child feeding was not
  included in the promotional messages

9.3   Too Much Space Between Bullets

Oftentimes, PowerPoint inserts substantial space between lines of text. This can
occur both as too much space between lines within a bullet as well as too much
space between bullets. All of this white space reduces the amount of space for communication and forces smaller font sizes that becomes difficult or impossible to
read, especially from the back of the room.

These spacing issues can be addressed by using the paragraph features of
PowerPoint. Set the line spacing to single, and make spacing before and after small
(e.g., <6 pt.). Another strategy to modify space between bullets is to insert a line
with a single letter of text. Color the text the same color as the background, and
adjust the font size to something small that optimizes spacing (Figs. 9.3.1, 9.3.2,
9.3.3, and 9.3.4).

Definitions and Data Analysis

- **Safe disposal**: Feces put/rinsed into latrine or specific pit or buried

- **Unsafe disposal**: Feces put/rinsed into drain or ditch/bush or jungle/garbage or left on the ground

- Compared characteristics of households with safe versus unsafe disposal of feces

- Generalized estimating equations to adjust for cluster design

Fig. 9.3.1 Lots of white space not well used that limits font size

Definitions

- **Safe disposal**: Feces put/rinsed into latrine or specific pit or buried
- **Unsafe disposal**: Feces put/rinsed into drain or ditch/bush or jungle/garbage or left on the ground

Data Analysis

- Compared characteristics of households with safe versus unsafe disposal of feces

- Generalized estimating equations to adjust for cluster design

Fig. 9.3.2 Reorganization of slide redistributes white space to better group and communicate ideas. Animation features could be used so that the top of the slide appear first and the data analysis section appears when the presenter clicks

Conclusions

- Restaurant staff and street food vendors in Bangladesh do not usually wash their hands with soap during food handling.

- Limited facilities contributes to a lack of hand and food hygiene

- Impractical for street food vendors to carry and store water

- Cost of soap is a barrier

Conclusions (2)

- Equated handwashing with hands contacting water

- Respondents perceived that customers are satisfied if they get tasty food

Fig. 9.3.3 So much space between the bullets that the list stretches across two slides

Conclusions

- Restaurant staff and street food vendors in Bangladesh do not usually wash their hands with soap during food handling.
- Limited facilities contributes to a lack of hand and food hygiene
- Impractical for street food vendors to carry and store water
- Cost of soap is a barrier
- Equated handwashing with hands contacting water
- Respondents perceived that customers are satisfied if they get tasty food

Fig. 9.3.4 Same bullets with reasonable spacing between fit on a single slide

9.4   Using Bullets Without Hanging Indents

Bullets help to format text so that it is clear there are a series of points. They improve readability of narrative. It is easiest to see the difference between points when a hanging indent is used on subsequent lines so that the separation between ideas is clear. In addition, a slightly larger spacing between points in contrast to lines within points further makes this separation easier to see and read (Figs. 9.4.1, 9.4.2 and 9.4.3).

•Antibiotic use has the potential to contribute to
antibiotic resistance
•Empiric prescription rates for mild respiratory illness
range from 40-60% in high-income countries.
•We reviewed icddr,b-IEDCR's collaborative hospital-
based influenza surveillance data collected from May
2007 to August 2014 to assess antibiotic prescriptions
for mild respiratory illness

Fig. 9.4.1 Bullets Without Hanging Indent (the Common Error)

• Antibiotic use has the potential to contribute to
  antibiotic resistance
• Empiric prescription rates for mild respiratory illness
  range from 40-60% in high-income countries.
• We reviewed icddr,b-IEDCR's collaborative hospital-
  based influenza surveillance data collected from May
  2007 to August 2014 to assess antibiotic prescriptions
  for mild respiratory illness

Fig. 9.4.2 Bullets with Hanging Indent

• Antibiotic use has the potential to contribute to antibiotic resistance

• Empiric prescription rates for mild respiratory illness range from 40-
  60% in high-income countries.

• We reviewed icddr,b-IEDCR's collaborative hospital-based influenza
  surveillance data collected from May 2007 to August 2014 to assess
  antibiotic prescriptions for mild respiratory illness

Fig. 9.4.3 Bullets with Hanging Indent, Single Space Within Points, with 1.2 Spaces Between Lines, and a More Horizontal Layout

9.5 Chart Junk

In his classic book, *The Visual Display of Quantitative Information*, Edward Tufte defines chart junk as visual elements in charts and graphs that are not necessary to comprehend the information represented, or that distract the viewer from this information. Among the worst promoters of chart junk are institutions that want all slides to have a common look that advertises the institution. These objectives run counter to clear communication. Clear communication will better promote a scientist and their institution's reputation compared with tacky backgrounds that obstruct and detract. Clear, large, and simple is the most effective pathway to clear visual communication. If your institution insists on a stylized template, we recommend using it only on the opening and closing slides (Figs. 9.5.1 and 9.5.2).

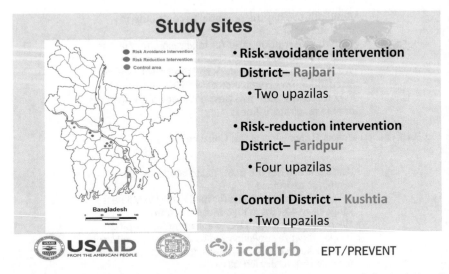

Fig. 9.5.1 A slide from a presentation using a template requested from the study funder designed to give credit to funders and a uniform look to the presentation

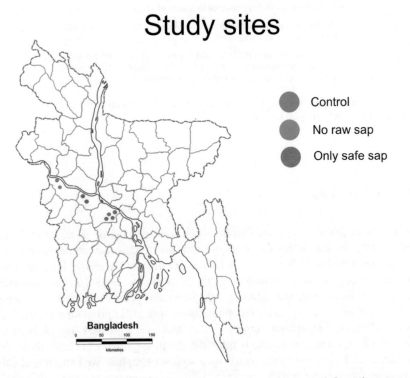

Fig. 9.5.2 A cleaner presentation of the slide with chart junk and extraneous information removed to permit attention to the key communication objectives

9.6   Using Three-Dimensional Chart Features as Decorations

Figures are used to connect to the visual centers of human perception and so improve communication of your quantitative results. Adding three dimensions to charts adds complexity. This complexity should only be invoked if it improves communication of the data. Otherwise, this three-dimensional imagery is chart junk (Error 9.5) that risk distracting the audience. Strive for minimalist elegant images that communicate without distraction (Figs. 9.6.1, 9.6.2, and 9.6.3).

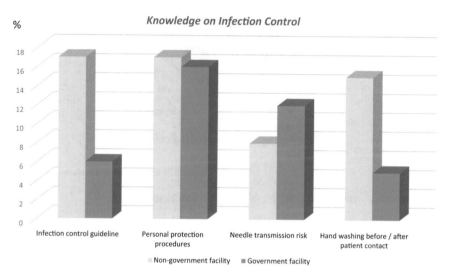

Fig. 9.6.1 Three dimensions used as uninformative chart junk

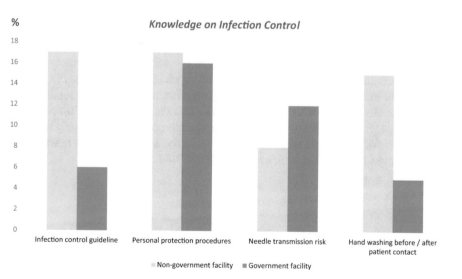

Fig. 9.6.2 Simpler cleaner chart

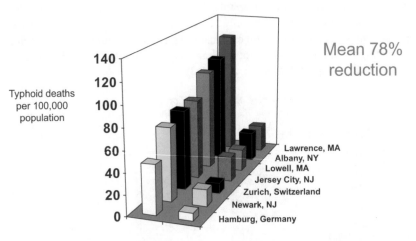

Fig. 9.6.3   Three-dimensional features used to support data communication

9.7   Using a Pie Chart

For a scientific presentation, simple pie charts are best avoided. It is safe to assume that a scientific audience understands percentage without having it illustrated. That is, they don't need an illustration to appreciate that 25% is one quarter of a pie.

Pie charts made using the default features of PowerPoint are particularly bad. In the PowerPoint pie chart, the reader has to jump back and forth between the pie and the legend to sort out what the particular proportion represents. This requirement that the reader decodes adds another cognitive task that detracts from simple communication. It invites the audience to focus attention on decoding your graphic at the expense of listening to what you are saying. If there is a compelling reason for a pie chart, use labeling that avoids a legend (Figs. 9.7.1 and 9.7.2).

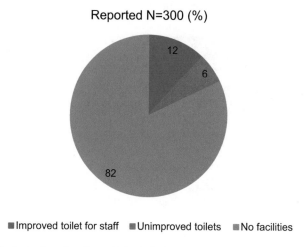

Fig. 9.7.1 Default pie chart from PowerPoint. It is both underinformative and requires decoding

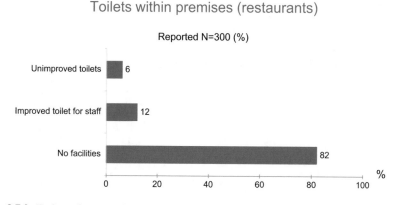

Fig. 9.7.2 Easier to interpret visualization of data from Fig. 9.16. The labels are right next to the numbers. No decoding required

An exception to the rule of avoiding a pie chart is when a comparison between two groups or a breakdown of a subgroup of a pie provides a useful illustration that engages the audience's visual understanding to interpret patterns in the data (Figs. 9.7.3 and 9.7.4).

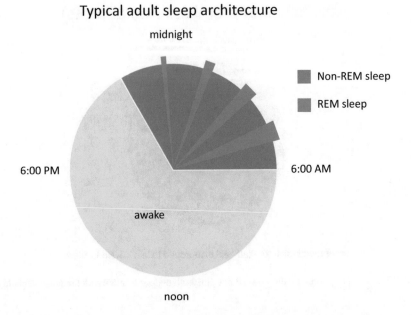

Fig. 9.7.3 An illustrative pie chart that effectively embeds additional meaning and communicates effectively

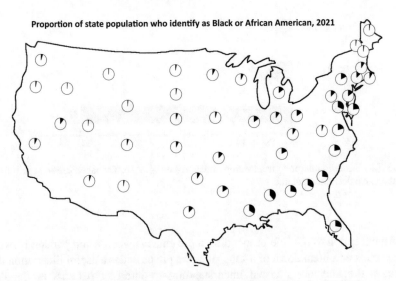

Fig. 9.7.4 A comparative pie chart that supports a visual understanding of a distribution

9.8 Using Vertical Bars When Horizontal Bars Would Communicate Better

Vertical bar charts are commonly used default formats in PowerPoint, but they are often not the best way to present data. If a useful description of the characteristic being presented is long, it is difficult to read in the constrained space or at an odd angle at the bottom of a slide. A horizontal bar allows more space and larger font to facilitate quick communication (Figs. 9.8.1, 9.8.2, and 9.8.3).

PowerPoint is quirky. In many versions of PowerPoint, the order of appearance of the horizontal bars is directly counterintuitive. That is, when you construct the data table, the first variable you enter displays at the bottom of the chart, and the bottom variable is at the top. You can simply reverse the order in the data table to have it present according to what aligns best with your communication objectives.

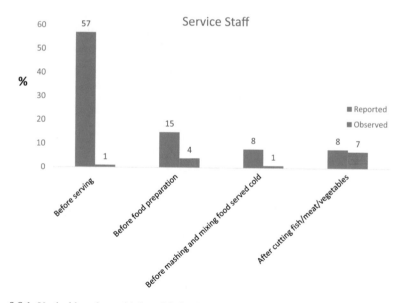

Fig. 9.8.1 Vertical bar chart with long labels. Note that the titles do not align intuitively with the bars. Our eyes are not accustomed to reading across odd angles

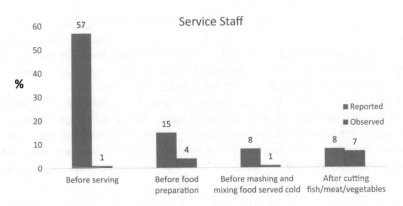

Fig. 9.8.2 Vertical bar chart with multiline descriptions. These are often small and difficult to read

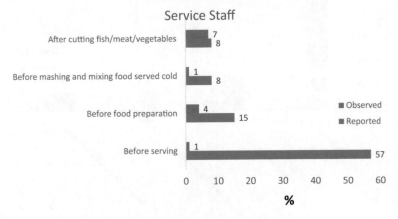

Fig. 9.8.3 Simpler, easier to read horizontal bar chart

9.9   Copying a Manuscript Figure Instead of Developing a Custom Figure

Constructing high-quality slides to support a verbal presentation requires considerable thought, creativity, and time. It might save time to use figures developed by others in your own presentation. Especially when you are reporting information from other research groups, it is quite tempting to copy directly from their manuscripts or, if you have access, to their slides. The drawback to this approach is that visual presentations used for one speaker in one context often have a somewhat different role in your own presentation. Copying and pasting someone else's work (even if appropriately attributed) is often not the best way to achieve your communication objective.

Each slide should be integrated with the narrative and communication objectives of your presentation and should be designed to help the audience succinctly understand your ideas. A visual presentation is quite different from reading a manuscript. Figures or tables in the manuscript can include more detail because the reader can take the time to work carefully through these details. By contrast, the pace of an oral presentation is quicker, and so the supporting information should be presented more simply in a clear format that the audience can intuitively grasp. If you find yourself saying "I apologize for the messiness of the slide, but I want to focus on this one issue . . ." or "This is hard to read, but. .. ," this is a message to yourself that the slide needs to be revised. Remove the messiness. Clearly communicate the one issue to the audience and jettison the apology (Figs. 9.9.1 and 9.9.2).

Country	n	HWWS after toilet (%)	HWWS after cleaning child (%)	HWWS after cleaning up child stools (%)	HWWS before feeding index child (%)
Ghana	500	3	2	—	1
Kerala, India	350	42	—	25	—
Madagascar	40	4	—	—	12
Kyrgyzstan	65	18	0	—	—
Senegal	450	23	18	—	—
Peru	500	14	—	—	6
Sichuan, China	78	13	—	16	6
Shaanxi, China	64	12	—	—	16
Tanzania	30	13	13[a]	13[a]	4
Uganda	500	14	19	11	6
Vietnam	720	—	14	23	5
Kenya[b]	802	29	35	38	13
Average		17	13	19	5

Curtis, V. et al, *Health Educ Res.* 2009 Aug;24(4):655-73.

Fig. 9.9.1 Slide developed by lifting a table from a manuscript

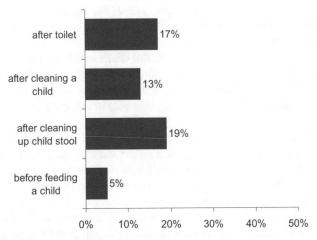

Handwashing with soap
structured observation, 11 country review
Sichuan, China; Shaanxi, China; Ghana; Kenya; Kerala, India; Kyrgyzstan; Madagascar; Peru; Senegal; Tanzania; Uganda; Vietnam

Fig. 9.9.2 Custom graphic derived from the table to communicate key messages to an audience. Note the elimination of most of the numbers, the removal of the confusing nonstandard abbreviation, yet noting the countries that were actually included

9.10   Photos with an Unnatural Aspect Ratio

Digital photography allows us to insert engaging photographs into our presentations. Often, to make the text fit more neatly with the photograph, we adjust the size of the photograph, but sometimes inadvertently we also affect the aspect ratio. The aspect ratio is the ratio of the width to the height. If the ratio of the width to the height is changed, the photograph appears distorted. This is particularly common when using PowerPoint and resizing the image by clicking and dragging. Below is the same photograph with three different aspect ratios (Figs. 9.10.1, 9.10.2, and 9.10.3).

Changing the aspect ratio distorts the picture and makes readers wonder whether the photographic subjects are oddly disproportioned. To make a photograph fit within a space, consider careful cropping and selecting the right size, but don't change the aspect ratio. You may also need a photograph with a different orientation. When combining text and photographs on a PowerPoint slide, vertically oriented photographs generally use the space better and are easier seen from the back of the room. Encourage your field team to compose photographic subjects that work well with a vertical orientation.

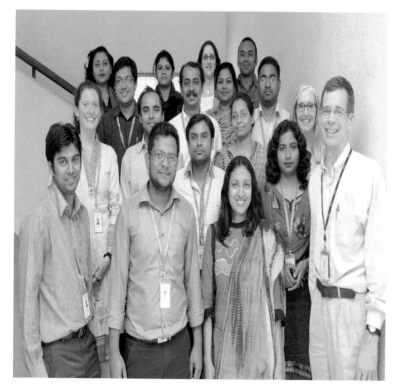

Fig. 9.10.1 The photographic subjects have been squeezed. That is, the horizontal aspect ratio is too small compared with the vertical

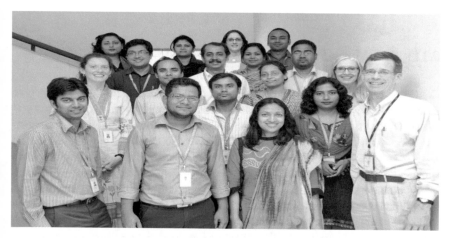

Fig. 9.10.2 Here the photograph has been stretched horizontally

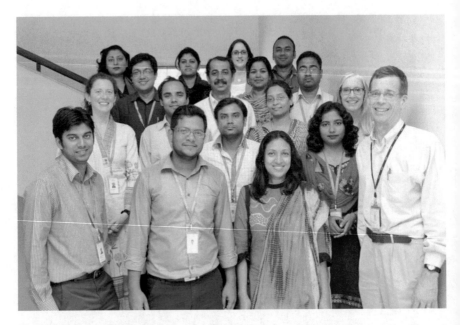

Fig. 9.10.3 This is the photograph as taken by the camera

One way to avoid distorted aspect ratios is to use the insert function on MS Word or MS PowerPoint to directly insert the file rather than using copy and paste. You can then adjust the size of the photograph by right-clicking on the photograph, select size and position, ensure that the "lock aspect ratio" box is checked, and then change the size of the photograph by incrementing the height or width using the arrow keys.

9.11   Too Many Photographs on a Single Slide

Context is critical for communicating public health scientific results. Many people in the audience will never have visited communities similar to where your study was conducted or understand the local practices and conditions. Photographs can communicate to an audience the situation that gave rise to the issue of public health interest and the people who are at risk through visual pathways that complement spoken description and written text.

A common saying asserts that a picture is worth 1000 words. Especially in an oral presentation when timing is strictly limited, an extra 1000 words to communicate your study is a huge asset. However, we would slightly modify the saying. That is, one good picture is worth 1000 words. A good picture illustrates your point and is easily seen by your audience. A plethora of pictures risks being distracting because they are too small to see by the half of your audience who are sitting in the back half of the room. Moreover, multiple pictures mean multiple messages, and so the audience may be focusing on trying to figure out what is in each of the tiny pictures, rather than listening to your verbal presentation (Figs. 9.11.1 and 9.11.2).

- **Data collection**:
- Respondent was a mother or caregiver of child under 5 yrs of age
- Measurements included:
  - Face-to-face interviews
  - Spot checks
  - Mid upper arm circumference
  - Hand washing demonstrations
- Data were collected in Smart phones/PDA

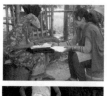
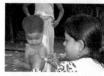
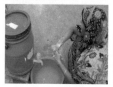

Fig. 9.11.1   Slide cluttered with too many photos

Study Participants

Mother or caregiver of child under 5 yr of age

Data collection

- Face-to-face interviews
- Spot checks
- Mid upper arm circumference
- Hand washing demonstrations

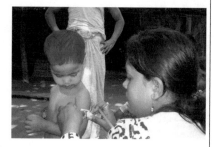

Fig. 9.11.2   The photograph is large enough that the audience can see the fieldworker measuring the child's upper arm

9.12 Fieldworkers as the Dominant Subject of Photographs

We cannot usually afford to include professional photographers on our field teams to capture images of the context where we work. Consequently, we depend upon fieldworkers or other members of the study team to take pictures that can be used to communicate context to our audience. Fieldworkers, however, are often particularly interested in pictures of the field team. Although this is occasionally a useful complement to a verbal presentation, photographs that illustrate the conditions as experienced by the target population are generally much more useful. We recommend specifying to the photographers on your team the photographic subjects that you are particularly interested in. Verbal presentations are often presented to audiences who have never been in the country or seen the conditions where the work was conducted, so photographs that provide an evocative illustration of these contexts are particularly useful to improve audience understanding (Figs. 9.12.1 and 9.12.2).

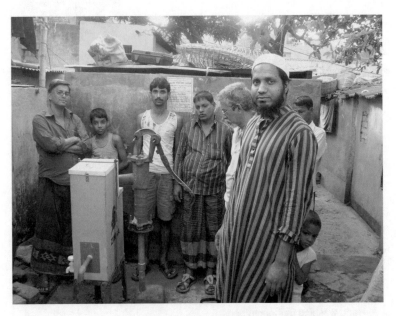

Fig. 9.12.1 Photograph of a water treatment device affixed to a hand pump surrounded by study personnel and men in the compound. This staged photograph displays involved workers, the device, and some information on context but does not show the device actually being used, nor does it include women who are the primary caretakers of household water

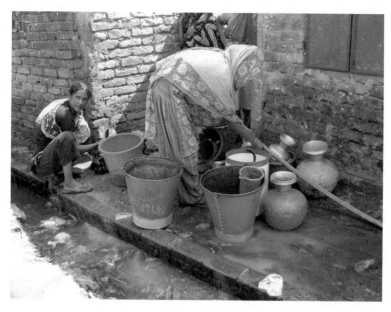

Fig. 9.12.2 This photograph shows women working with a compromised water supply near an open drain. It illustrates the cramped surrounding and the proximity of supply water to contamination

9.13   Including a Final "Thank You" Slide

Having your final slide say "Thank You" (presumably to the audience for their attention), often accompanied by an illustration that is irrelevant to the theme of your talk, is common in some contexts. Such slides are less common in an international scientific forum. Indeed, they often appear out of place. The gratuitous graphics distract from the major communication message of your talk. Drop such slides. Your final slide should either be acknowledgments or conclusions (Fig. 9.13.1).

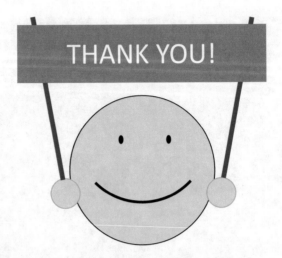

Fig. 9.13.1 A final "Thank You" slide should be left out of the presentation

9.14   Failure to Separate Ideas in a Multilined Title

When typing a sentence, after producing sufficient text to fill a line, the next word appears on the next line. This works fine for sentences but is suboptimal for titles. Titles are an integral element of the visual presentation of your ideas. By thoughtfully dividing the title into natural parts, the audience can more quickly understand your message (Figs. 9.14.1, 9.14.2, 9.14.3, and 9.14.4).

**Phase 1: Identifying the Barriers to Fecal
Sludge Management**

Fig. 9.14.1   Multiline title running to the end of the line

**Phase 1: Identifying the Barriers
to Fecal Sludge Management**

Fig. 9.14.2   Better title split by ideas

**How do street food vendors access toilet
facilities?**

Fig. 9.14.3   Default splitting of title

**How do street food vendors
access toilet facilities?**

Fig. 9.14.4   Improved title with ideas grouped together

Open Access   This chapter is licensed under the terms of the Creative Commons Attribution 4.0 International License (http://creativecommons.org/licenses/by/4.0/), which permits use, sharing, adaptation, distribution and reproduction in any medium or format, as long as you give appropriate credit to the original author(s) and the source, provide a link to the Creative Commons license and indicate if changes were made.

The images or other third party material in this chapter are included in the chapter's Creative Commons license, unless indicated otherwise in a credit line to the material. If material is not included in the chapter's Creative Commons license and your intended use is not permitted by statutory regulation or exceeds the permitted use, you will need to obtain permission directly from the copyright holder.

Appendix 1
Concept Note Outline

1. Title of the proposed study
2. Objective(s)

    (a) What key knowledge will the study generate?

3. Background

    (a) Current state of knowledge on specific study question

       (i) Not a general review but tightly focused on study question
      (ii) Cite key literature

    (b) Specify the gap in current knowledge
    (c) Describe the relevance of the study question. Why should readers/funders care?

4. Methods

    (a) Study site and study population
    (b) Study design
    (c) Key definitions (e.g., case definitions)
    (d) Sampling methods
    (e) Data collection process
    (f) Laboratory analysis
    (g) Primary and secondary outcome variables
    (h) Analytical plan
    (i) Sample size assumptions and calculation
    (j) Collaborators

© The Editor(s) (if applicable) and The Author(s) 2022
S. Luby, D. L. Southern, *The Pathway to Publishing: A Guide to Quantitative Writing in the Health Sciences*, https://doi.org/10.1007/978-3-030-98175-4

(k) Ethical considerations

(l) Limitations

5. Timeline

   (a) Gantt chart

6. Budget

   (a) Construct this using an intuitive format that you can revise as the study design, and sample size is further developed.
   (b) Estimate unit costs of personnel and supplies for an initial draft. Clarify costs in subsequent versions.

Appendix 2
Concept Note Example

Temporal Variability of Chlorine Demand in Dhaka, Bangladesh

By Fred Goddard

Study Question

What is the temporal variability in chlorine consumption by inorganic and organic materials in water, both daily and seasonally, in the piped water supply system of Dhaka, Bangladesh? How does this affect the type of chlorination injection systems required to continuously provide water with a minimum chlorine residual of 0.2 mg/l, congruent with WHO standards, for safe drinking water?

Objectives

The goal of this study is to better understand how the effectiveness of chlorination methods at the point of distribution, point of collection, or point of use is affected by temporal variability in chlorine demand (chlorine that has been added to water and is consumed by organic and inorganic matter in the water) by:

1. Assessing the daily patterns and variability of chlorine demand.
2. Assessing the impact of rainfall events and temperature on chlorine demand by compiling chlorine demand data in Dhaka's three weather seasons: summer, monsoon, and winter.
3. Generate hypotheses for major contributors to elevated chlorine demand, such as power outages or increased water residence time, that could help manage spikes in chlorine demand across water points.

© The Editor(s) (if applicable) and The Author(s) 2022
S. Luby, D. L. Southern, *The Pathway to Publishing: A Guide to Quantitative Writing in the Health Sciences*, https://doi.org/10.1007/978-3-030-98175-4

Rationale

Lack of access to safe drinking water is estimated to cause 23% of deaths by diarrheal diseases among children under the age of 5 in South Asia (C Boschi-Pinto 2009). Dhaka is one of the most densely populated cities in South Asia, with over 50,000 people per square mile, and approximately one-third of its residents live in slums (G Angeles 2009). A 2010 survey conducted by the Lotus Water team at the International Centre for Diarrhoeal Disease Research, Bangladesh, found that 80% of randomly selected samples of 127 slum water points in Dhaka were contaminated with *E. coli*. The primary reasons for unsafe water in Dhaka, which is mostly pumped from central groundwater pumping stations, are considered to be the leaky, intermittently pressurized water distribution systems, a common issue not only in Dhaka but throughout Asia with over half of its water supply shown to be intermittent (van den Berg 2011). In addition, high temperatures and severe weather events, particularly during the monsoon season, typically affect the quality of the drinking water negatively (Mirza 2007). The challenges faced in Dhaka due to the nature of the water supply infrastructure, the limited capacity and resources available to the municipality, as well as the difficult weather conditions are challenges encountered by many other urban areas in South Asia (UN 1987).

Chlorination is widely considered to be one of the more cost-effective water disinfection methods to provide water that is safe for consumption (Water Quality & Health Council 2003). In Dhaka, it is being implemented at the point of distribution via chlorine injection pumps as well as at the point of use with chlorine tablets. In addition, the Lotus Water team (www.lotuswater.org) is piloting an automatic chlorination device that disinfects the water at the point of collection, for example, at shared hand pumps and shared water points. Regardless at what stage the water is disinfected, it is desirable to not only have sufficient amount of chlorine in the water to kill pathogens but to also have a residual amount of chlorine, specified as a minimum of 0.2 mg/L by the World Health Organization, to ensure the water is safe in storage and stop it from becoming recontaminated. The total chlorine residual in a sample of water is influenced by the dose of chlorine added and the chlorine demand of the water, which is the chlorine that reacts first with inorganic and organic materials in the water and is thus not available for disinfection (CDC 2014).

However, it is necessary to dose accurately and not significantly exceed this minimum because the taste and odor of chlorinated water becomes unacceptable at high dosing, particularly in settings where the populations are not regularly exposed to chlorinated drinking water (Flanagan 2013). We recently conducted a pilot study in Dhaka to determine a threshold of chlorine concentration at which the water becomes unacceptable to drink to local communities. Our preliminary data suggests that this threshold lies between 0.8 mg/L and 1 mg/L. Subsequently, chlorine demand presents a particular challenge to this context because there is a fine line in dosing enough chlorine to exceed the minimum of 0.2 mg/l but stay below the threshold of 0.8–1 mg/L. As a result, to be able to ensure that an adequate and acceptable dose of chlorine is added, so that the water is continuously fully disinfected and safe in storage as well as being of acceptable taste and odor, it is important to understand the nature of chlorine demand in Dhaka's water supply system.

In August 2014, we conducted a study pilot to compare the spatial distribution of chlorine demand between 18 water samples collected in four different slums in central Dhaka. This pilot allowed us to develop a method to best collect water samples in Dhaka and detect chlorine demand in the sampled raw water. To find the chlorine demand, it is the chlorine residual 30 minutes after the manual addition of chlorine (WHO 1996) in each water sample that is measured, which is the remaining chlorine that is available for disinfection in storage. The chlorine residual from identical doses of chlorine between chlorine demand free water, for example, distilled water, is compared to a raw water sample that has been collected from at a water point in Dhaka. This is further outlined in the data collection section.

Chlorine demand can vary over time in Dhaka because of water use patterns and inconsistent pumping regimes caused by electricity cuts, causing fluctuating pressures and residence times in the system. Low pressure and high residence times are conducive to an increased infiltration of organic and inorganic matter into the leaky piped water system, leading to reduced water quality and hence increased chlorine demand. In addition, weather conditions that vary daily but especially seasonally, such as temperature and rainfall events, have an impact on water quality in South Asia (Abdul Hussain Shar 2008) and Bangladesh (MOEF 2001). Microbiological quality of the water is negatively impacted by the addition of organic and inorganic matter, and changes in water quality affect chlorine demand.

Finally, it is important not only to gain a better understanding of temporal chlorine demand patterns but also to generate hypotheses for the primary causes of spikes in chlorine demand to be able to better predict elevations in chlorine demand without having to frequently take measurements. Chlorine demand is affected not only by differences in water quality caused by local conditions but also by changes in water quality caused by low pressure and high residence times commonly found in an intermittent water supply system (E Kumpel 2013). This study will help gain a better understanding of the causes of chlorine demand, as well as its temporal variability, which will guide future decisions on what chlorine injection technologies are appropriate and effective.

Outcomes and Exposures

Primary Outcome
Total chlorine demand in water samples collected in Dhaka is the primary outcome variable measured by this study. It is a continuous variable that will be measured with our previously developed chlorine demand detection method, which will be described further in the data collection section.

Secondary Outcome

Our hypotheses for spikes in chlorine demand will be tested, and additional hypotheses will be generated through qualitative research outlined in the study design section.

Primary Exposures

The primary exposures that can influence different water quality parameters, which in turn affect chlorine consumption, are external events such as pump outages due to power cuts, high residence times due to low water demand, or rain events during the monsoon season. Other exposures have so far not been considered for this study but will be identified during the qualitative research component described under objective 3 in the study design section. Exposures will not be measured but rather identified by examining existing records for the relevant exposures and comparing those to chlorine demand measurements taken in the field. For example, DWASA (Dhaka Water and Sewerage Authority) have records on pump outages, and weather data can be pulled from weather reports.

Secondary Exposures

During our study pilot of 18 water points in Dhaka, we aimed to confirm what we hypothesized to be the primary drivers for chlorine consumption in Dhaka's piped water supply. We tested for iron, manganese, turbidity, and flow rate. Our results showed that there was no statistically significant correlation between any of these exposures and levels of chlorine demand. As a result of our findings from the study pilot, this study is not designed to conduct further work to identify the exposures in the water quality for chlorine consumption in Dhaka's water. Approximately 30% of the resources for the study pilot were used to measure these exposures, and it is not considered to be the most effective and relevant use of funds for the study in temporal variability.

Study Design

To fulfill objectives 1–3, the most appropriate approach identified is a combination of two study designs. A nonexperimental exposed cohort study will fulfill objectives 1 and 2 by taking chlorine demand measurements at water points and analyzing them for variability. We can assume that all water points are exposed to some organic or inorganic matter, leading to chlorine demand. To fulfill objective 3, a case review study design will be employed. This will be accomplished by using chorine demand data that has been gathered to fulfill objectives 1 and 2 and comparing that to hypotheses generated for exposures found in the qualitative research component of this study. This qualitative research will be conducted retrospectively by questioning water point users on the water quality as well as accessing publicly available data on hypothesized causality for spikes in chlorine demand.

Objective 1: To fulfill this objective, water samples shall be collected two times daily with consideration to DWASA's water use data. For example, the first sample shall be collected after the longest period of low water demand, typically early in the morning. The second sample shall be collected after the longest period of peak demand, typically in the late afternoon/early evening. Should water not be available at the time of collection, the water samples shall be collected as soon as steady-state conditions are reached once the pumps come back on line.

Objective 2: There are three seasons in Bangladesh. A hot and humid summer from March to June, a milder and wet monsoon season from June to October, and a cool and dry winter from October to March. Water samples as outlined in objective 1 shall be collected during all three seasons. The summer data shall be collected during the first and last week in April, the monsoon data in the first and last week in July, and the winter data in the first and last week in January. The data collected in each of these months for each water point and for each time period (morning and afternoon/evening) shall be compared to weather data for each day that samples have been collected.

Objective 3: To fulfill the final objective, the quantitative data collected shall be compared to qualitative data collected retrospectively on reasons outlined for poor water quality by local users as well as the previously hypothesized causality (high residence times, pump system failures, and monsoon rains). This qualitative data will be collected using two methods. During each water sample collection, compound members will be asked about any changes in water quality since the previous collection using a questionnaire. For example, if a data collector visits a water point on a Tuesday morning for sample collection, he/she will inquire to water point users about any notable changes in water quality or other events relating to the water (e.g., no water available, low pressure) since Monday evening's visit. In addition, data will be gathered from available local information on our hypothesized causality for chlorine demand. For example, DWASA reports on pump failures, external weather reports on heavy rainfall events, and correspondence with the DWASA operators responsible for pump stations shall be compared to the relevant time periods of chlorine demand data collected.

Analysis

Objective 1: The primary analysis will begin by finding the ranges in chlorine demand for every water point on a daily basis in a given season. It is the distribution of these ranges we are particularly interested in because it is distribution rather than the absolute values of chlorine demand that will present the greatest challenge to effective continuous chlorination. If the absolute value of chlorine demand is comparatively high, but there is no significant difference over time, chlorine injection technologies can account for this by continuously adding a higher dose of chlorine, providing the remains acceptable to drink for taste and odor. If there is high variability, current technologies might not be able to continuously ensure a chlorine residual in the water without a difficult-to-implement, complex treatment algorithm. By finding the ranges in chlorine demand, we can understand to what extent we might be able to add a sufficient amount of chlorine to the water. To investigate the ranges for every water point, the maximum value for chlorine demand is subtracted by the minimum value for each day.

Objective 2: For objective 2, we would primarily compare chlorine demand measurements immediately before and after major weather events, whether these spread across several days or are just on a single day. Chlorine demand data will be collected over two different sets of days for each season, during the first and last week in January, April, and July, respectively. In addition, we will compare the distribution of ranges between the three seasons to paint a more general picture of differences arising from overall varying conditions.

Objective 3: For the final objective, the measured data for each water point will be analyzed in comparison to data collected through our qualitative research on perceived causality for low water quality by water point users as well as major external events (such as weather or system failures) to generate hypotheses for spikes in chlorine demand. The questionnaire used for interviews of water point users shall be analyzed using a combination of a priori (such as "low pressure" and "no water available") codes and emergent codes. Answers to this questionnaire shall be coded by the person running the chlorine demand study with extensive knowledge on causality for low water quality and how this relates to chlorine demand since some of the reasoning for changes in water quality provided by the users might not be reasons supported by scientific evidence.

Study Sample

Target Population
Urban water points in low- and middle-income countries used for household purposes, such as drinking and cooking, supplied by a piped distribution system.

Study Population
Shared water points in the slums of Dhaka, Bangladesh, supplied by the local municipal piped distribution system.

Sampling Method
The sampling for this study shall be conducted with a multistage sampling method where a set of water points shall be chosen from different clusters for purposive sampling. Each cluster represents a different set of water points that are supplied by the same central municipal groundwater pumping station. The chosen clusters must have daily water supply data for their respective pumping stations available. Water points in each cluster shall be chosen systematically but must meet the criteria outlined below:

- Shared water point
- Connected to the DWASA piped distribution system
- Distribution system shall be supplied by one of DWASA's deep groundwater tube wells
- Water point shall be accessible at all times during the day, from early in the morning to late in the evening
- Owner of water point must agree to two 4-day period of sample collection during the first and last week in January, April, and July, respectively.

Sample Size

The sample size was determined with a focus on gathering enough samples to fulfill objective 1. However, this sample size will have to be big enough to allow for changes in weather conditions in a given season to fulfill objective 2. Since objective 3 is a hypothesis-generating rather than a hypothesis testing exercise, the sample size will not be influenced by this objective. The primary outcome variable measured to fulfill objectives 1 and 2 is the level of chlorine demand in samples drawn from shared water points connected to the municipal piped water system in Dhaka. The sample size will have to allow for an analysis that shows if there are differences in chlorine demand in a given day and what those differences are. We hypothesize that samples collected in the morning before daily water use has established itself will have higher chlorine demand than samples in the afternoon and evening during peak water use. So the underlying question is: **How many water points do we need to access twice a day to show the anticipated intra-daily differences in chlorine demand?**

No published findings were identified that show variations in chlorine demand in water distribution systems comparable to Dhaka. The difference in the means and standard deviations for the morning versus evening sample utilized for this sample size calculation is an estimate formulated from our previous experience with water quality research in Dhaka and our chlorine demand pilot study. Sample 1 outlined in Table A1 is the morning sample and sample 2 the evening sample.

The first two iterations (even at a nonstandard power of 0.9) showed a smaller sample size than anticipated because of the high difference between morning and evening samples (0.4 ppm) and low standard deviations that were assumed. The next iterations were performed with a smaller difference between the two sample means at 0.3 ppm. The two sample means, 0.5 ppm and 0.8 ppm, are in line with our chlorine demand pilot where we found a mean of 0.64 ppm chlorine demand for water points that were tested at various times during the day. The standard deviations were chosen to allow for a distribution with chlorine demand values closer to zero as well as values above 1 ppm. As comparison, the standard deviation during our 18 water point study pilot was 0.27 ppm, in line with our standard deviations for the final two sample calculations. A design effect of 1.8 was chosen to account for

Table A1 Iterations of sample size calculations

Sample 1 mean	Sample 1 standard deviation	Sample 2 mean	Sample 2 standard deviation	Confidence interval	Power	Sample ratio	Design effect	Sample size[a]
0.8	0.25	0.4	0.1	95%	80%	1:1	1.8	**16**
0.8	0.25	0.4	0.1	95%	90%	1:1	1.8	**18**
0.8	0.25	0.5	0.15	95%	90%	1:1	1.8	**36**
0.8	0.35	0.5	0.25	95%	80%	1:1	1.8	**60**
0.8	0.35	0.5	0.25	95%	90%	1:1	1.8	**78**

[a]Sample size is given as "Total Sample Size," so a sample size of 16 would equal eight water points where two water samples are collected daily

clustering—water points are divided into clusters where each cluster represents a set of water points that is supplied by the same groundwater pumping station and the same distribution network. Power of 0.9 is not considered to be necessary for this type of study, so the penultimate iteration was chosen to determine the sample size for this study.

This leads to a sample size of 60, which amounts to 30 water points. Using eight water points across four clusters will fulfill this sample size and total 32 water points for sample collection. Sample collectors will rotate the order in which water points are accessed for sample collection, that is, by accessing water points in order 12345678 on day one, 23456781 on day two, 34567812 on day three, and so on. This will require 8 days of sampling—4 days at the beginning of each month and 4 days at the end of each month—to ensure samples have been collected in all orders.

Data Collection

The primary measurements required for this study are chlorine consumption in water samples collected at Dhaka's water points.

Strategy
Water samples will have to be collected in the field and be processed in the lab the same day. Eight 0.5 L water samples will fit into a standard cooler (water can be stored at 4 °C for up to 24 hours (WHO 1996)). One cooler can be carried through a cluster by the data collector to collect all samples and can be transported back to the office via local public transportation. Water shall be sampled twice a day at each water point. The morning sampling for each cluster shall begin 2 hours before domestic water demand establishes itself, for example, from 5 to 7 am, since our previous work on collecting water samples in Dhaka suggested a maximum of 15 minutes for each sample, which will total to 2 hours of sampling. The sampling at all four clusters shall begin at a time relevant to their respective water supply data. Each cluster will require a different data collector as much of the sampling will be carried out simultaneously. After the first sample collection, the sample collector shall fill out the brief questionnaire outlined below:

- Compound name
- Location
- Site Nr
- DWASA tube well
- Connection legal or illegal
- Type of connection (flex. pipe, direct to main line, tank connected to main line)

Collection at the same water points shall be repeated in the late afternoon/evening for all 32 water points across the four clusters during 2 hours of peak demand. As outlined previously, sample collectors shall rotate the order in which water points are accessed for sample collection on a daily basis. After every sample collection, the sample collector shall fill out a questionnaire prompting the users of the tested water point on any issues with the water since the last visit:

- Have you experienced anything different with your water, such as taste, odor, color, or flow rate, since our last visit on [day] at [time]?
- If yes, can you please describe what these differences were?
- Where do you think these differences may come from?

In addition, each water sample shall be labeled as outlined below:

- Name of collector
- Site Nr.
- Date
- Time

After the eight samples have been collected, they shall be delivered to the lab for testing immediately.

Chlorine Detection

Our previous work on chlorine demand in Dhaka has allowed us to develop a method to best detect chlorine demand in Dhaka's raw water in the laboratory. To find the total chlorine consumed by organic and inorganic matter, it is the chlorine residual after manual addition of chlorine in each water sample we are analyzing, which is the remaining chlorine that is available for disinfection in storage. The chlorine residual from identical doses of chlorine between chlorine demand free water, for example, distilled water, is compared to a raw water sample that has been collected from a water point in Dhaka. For example, if you introduce 1.5 mg of sodium hypochlorite in the form of locally available liquid bleach in to a 0.5 L sample of distilled water, you would expect to have a chlorine concentration of 3 ppm (or 3 mg/L) in the chlorine demand free water. However, if you introduce the same amount of sodium hypochlorite into raw water, you might get a chlorine concentration of 2 ppm. This would mean that the inorganic and organic matter present in the water have consumed 1 ppm of chlorine, which in turn means the raw water has a chlorine demand of 1 ppm. A more detailed protocol for this sample collection in the field and measurements taken in the lab is outlined in Appendix 1.

Human Subjects

Institutional Review Boards will review the protocol for this study for human subject consideration at Stanford University and at the International Centre for Diarrhoeal Disease Research, Bangladesh. While this study does not influence its human subjects directly through an intervention, data collectors will have to enter slum compounds and access water points shared by households twice a day during the 8 days allocated for each season, thus impacting people's daily routines and needs. In addition, data collectors will be briefly interviewing a compound member during each visit as outlined in the data collection section.

Informed consent will be collected from water point owners, typically compound landlords (compounds in Dhaka are typically shared between 5 and 50 households in Dhaka). Water point owners must consent to two sample collections over 4-day periods during the first and last week in January, April, and July, respectively.

Informed consent will also be collected from compound members before the short interview at sample collection. Water point owners and interviewees will not be compensated.

Collaboration

This study will be conducted in collaboration between Stanford University and the International Centre for Diarrhoeal Disease Research, Bangladesh (icddr,b). It will build on a multiyear relationship between the two institutions while leveraging the resources of the Lotus Water project team. Lotus Water was established 4 years ago as a partnership between icddr,b and Stanford. The project is developing community-based water disinfection devices for shared water points to provide safe water to Dhaka's slums. We have faculty and students based at Stanford and an eight-person strong field team based in Dhaka. This study will build on the capacity and experience of our team in water quality and chlorination research in Dhaka's slums. Our field assistants in Dhaka were trained on data collection during our chlorine demand study pilot, and we have two field research assistants to help manage our field team. Our principal investigators, research associate, and graduate students frequently travel to Dhaka for other project work.

Timeline and Budget

The anticipated duration for this study is 23 months, and it will cost $66,500. A timeline is outlined in Appendix 2 and the budget in Appendix 3. The budget and timeline were developed, taking into consideration that our team has already built the capacity at icddr,b in Dhaka. This study will run in parallel to our other project work, and as a result, the gaps in data collection that are shown on the timeline are not a concern for the graduate students or the field assistants that will help with data collection.

Limitations

There are several limitations and weaknesses to the proposed study design that are worth noting:

- **Purposive sampling**: From the sample size generated for this study, we will not have the power to draw a purely representative sample for temporal variability in chlorine demand in Dhaka, but we will be able to gain an understanding for the extent of a challenge temporal variability in chlorine demand may present to chlorine injection systems.
- **Clustering**: A multistage sampling method was chosen for this study with four clusters that each represent a set of water points supplied by the same groundwa-

ter pumping station and distribution system. Even with the design effect added to the sample size calculations, there will be clustering in the chlorine demand data because the water points are being supplied from the same source and are supplied by the same piped system. However, the clustering of water points is necessary to reduce travel time and allow sample collectors to gather data in the 2-hour window described previously.

- **Causality:** The qualitative research for this study is designed as a hypothesis-generating exercise. As a result, it will not be possible to conclude causal relationships between the hypotheses generated and spikes in chlorine demand.

References

Hussain Shar, Yasmeen Faiz Kazi and Irshad Hussain Soomro. "Impact of Seasonal Variation on Bacteriological Quality of Drinking Water." *Bangladesh Journal of Microbiology*, 2008: 69–72.

C Boschi-Pinto, L Velebit, K Shibuya. "Estimating child mortality due to diarrhoea in developing countries." *Bulletin of the World Health Organization* 86 (2009): 710–717.

CDC. *Centers for Disease Control and Prevention: The Safe Water System.* 2014. http://www.cdc.gov/safewater/chlorine-residual-testing.html (accessed January 2015).

Dean, A., K. Sullivan, and M Soe. *OpenEpi: Open Source Epidemiologic Statistics for Public Health.* 9 22, 2014. www.OpenEpi.com (accessed 2 23, 2015).

E Kumpel, K Nelson. "Comparing microbial water quality in an intermittent and continuous piped water supply." *Water Research* 37 (2013): 5176–5188.

Flanagan, S. Meng, X. and Zheng Y. "Increasing acceptance of chlorination for household water treatment: observations from Bangladesh." *Waterlines* 32, no. 2 (2013): 125–134.

G Angeles, P Lance, J Bardon-O'Fallon, N Islam, A Mahbub, N I Nazem. "The 2005 census and mapping of slums in Bangladesh: design, select results and application." *International Journal of Health Geographics* 32 (2009): 1–19.

Mirza, M. *Climate Change, Adaptation and Adaptive Governance in Water Sector in South Asia.* Toronto: Adaptation and Impacts Research Division - Environment Canada, 2007, 1–19.

MOEF. *Bangladesh: The State of the Environment.* Dhaka: Ministry of Environment and Forest Bangladesh, 2001.

UN. *Report of the World Commission on Environment and Development: Our Common Future.* New York City: WCED, 1987.

van den Berg, C. and Danilenko, A. *The IBENET Water Supply and Sanitation Performance Blue Book.* Washington, DC: World Bank, 2011.

Water Quality & Health Council. "Drinking Water Chlorination: A Review of Disinfection Practices and Issues." 2003.

WHO. *Guidelines for Drinking-Water Quality.* Geneva: World Health Organization, 1996.

WHO. *Water Quality Monitoring – A Practical Guide to the Design and Implementation of Freshwater Quality Studies and Monitoring Programmes.* Nairobi/Geneva: UNEP/WHO, 1996.

Timeline

Task	May	Jun	Jul	Aug	Sep	Oct	Nov	Dec	Jan	Feb	Mar	Apr	May	Jun	Personnel
Protocol Development*		█													PI, RA, GS
Stanford University approval				█											PI, RA, GS
ICDDR,B approval				█											PI, RA, GS
Finalize contract with ICDDR,B**					█										PI, RA, GS
Hire local field team**						█									RA, GS
Train local field team**							█								GS, FRA, FA
Survey water points that meet criteria							█								GS, FRA, FA
Winter sample collection and measurements								█							GS, FRA, FA
Preliminary winter quantative data clean up and analysis									█						GS
Winter qualitative data analysis (Objective 3)										█					FRA, GS
Summer sample collection and measurements											█				GS, FRA, FA
Preliminary summer quantative data clean up and analysis												█			GS
Summer qualitative data analysis (Objective 3)													█		FRA, GS
Monsoon sample collection and measurements						█									GS, FRA, FA
Preliminary monsoon quantative data clean up and analysis							█								GS
Monsoon qualitative data analysis (Objective 3)								█							FRA, GS
Full quantative data analysis (Objective 1 & 2)									█						GS
Manuscript - First draft										█					GS
Manuscript review by co-authors (first draft)											█				PI, RA
Manuscript - Second draft											█				GS
Manuscript review by co-authors (second draft)												█			PI, RA
Manuscript submission												█			GS
Manuscript review													█		
Manuscript revision and re-submission														█	PI, RA, GS

* Assuming I have funding by June - Timeline would be shifted depending on when funding comes in (Data collection may begin in a different season)

** This is arguably somewhat conservative, since I am assuming I will need a new team. We already have a field team who I trained in chlorine demand water sampling during the pilot study.

Personnel Key:		Time (months)
PI = Principe Investigator		8
RA = Research Associate		9
GS = Graduate Student		21
FRA = Field Research Assistant		9
FA = Field Assistant		6

Budget

Budget

Stanford University Budget

Personell	Quantity		Cost ($/month)	Time (Months)		Percent time (%)	Total cost
Research Associate	1		7500	6		8	3600
Graduate Student	1		6250	15		32	30000
					Total		33600.00

Travel	Quantity	Unit Cost	Total Cost	
International flights	1	2000	2000	Trip from Dec-Aug for all work in Dhaka.
Visa	1	160	160	
		Total (40%)	864	Study will only take on 40% of this cost, because that is how much time student will spend working on the project while in Dhaka (based on timeline)

Transport	Study Days	Cost ($/day)	Total Cost
Student	96	2.50	240
		Total	240

Lodging	Months	Cost ($/month)	Total Cost	
Dhaka student apartment	12	500	6000	
Student services fee	12	41.67	500	
		Total (0%)	0	(Lodging is included in graduate student stipend)

Per diem	Days	Cost ($/day)	Total Cost	
Daily expenses	225	15	3375	
		Total (0%)	0	(Per diem is included in graduate student stipend)

Overhead	Items charged to overhead	Cost	Overhead* %	Total cost
Stanford	Salaries, Travel, Transport	34704.00	60.5	20995.92
			Total	20995.92

*For federal funding sources

Stanford cost ($)	55700

ICDDR,B Budget

Personell	Quantity	Cost ($/month)	Time (Months)	Percent time (%)	Total cost
Field Research Assisstant	1	461	7	30	968.10
Field Assisstant	3	225.00	4	60	1620.00
				Total	2588

Transport	Study Days	Cost ($/day)	Total Cost	
FA & FRA	186	2		372
		Total		372

Equipment	Quantity	Unit cost ($)	Total Cost	
Lamotte Colorimeter	1	400		400
DPD liquid reagents	4	6		24
Sample collection bottles	24	1.80		43.16
Glass testing bottles	24	2.04		48.86
Liquid bleach	3	2.50		7.50
		Total		524

Overhead	Cost	Overhead %	Total cost	
Salaries, Transport	2960.10	30		888.03
		Total		888

ICDDRB cost ($)   4372

Total Cost $60072

Appendix 3
Critical Questions for Protocol Development

Thinking Critically

1. What is your overall research question?
2. What is the hypothesis that you want to test?
3. What is the aim(s) of your study?
4. What do scientists already know about the subject?
5. What do n'tscientists know about the subject (the gap in knowledge)?
6. Why i s this research important? What kind of answers will the study provide?

Research Design and Methods

7. Whom will you study?
8. What type of study design will you use to test your hypothesis?
9. What is your sample size?
10. How did you estimate your sample size?
11. What is the statistical power of your study?
12. How did you select your study unit of population (explain sampling method)?
13. How will you collect your data?

Data Analysis

14. What variables will you assess?

   (a) Outcome variables
   (b) Exposure variables

15. How will you measure these variables?

   (a) For categorical variables, what are the category definitions?

16. How will you analyze your data to test your hypothesis?

© The Editor(s) (if applicable) and The Author(s) 2022
S. Luby, D. L. Southern, *The Pathway to Publishing: A Guide to Quantitative Writing in the Health Sciences*, https://doi.org/10.1007/978-3-030-98175-4

Ethics

17. How will you protect human/animal rights?

Logistics

18. How long will the study take? What is your timeline?
19. How much will this cost?
20. When will the results become available, and how will you disseminate them?

Appendix 4
Framing Document

Title of paper:

Objective(s) of the paper:

Main result(s)

1.

2.

3.

Tables, figures or graphs that support your main results:

(Example only....you might have 5 tables, or any combination)

Table 1:

Table 2:

Figure 1:

Figure 2:

Table 3:

© The Editor(s) (if applicable) and The Author(s) 2022
S. Luby, D. L. Southern, *The Pathway to Publishing: A Guide to Quantitative
Writing in the Health Sciences*, https://doi.org/10.1007/978-3-030-98175-4

Appendix 5
Flowchart for Review of Scientific Documents

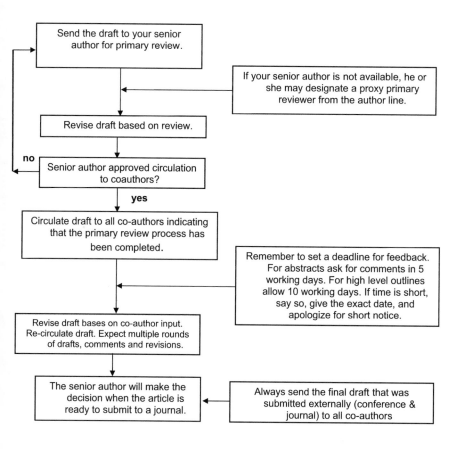

Send the draft to your senior author for primary review.

If your senior author is not available, he or she may designate a proxy primary reviewer from the author line.

Revise draft based on review.

no

Senior author approved circulation to coauthors?

yes

Circulate draft to all co-authors indicating that the primary review process has been completed.

Remember to set a deadline for feedback. For abstracts ask for comments in 5 working days. For high level outlines allow 10 working days. If time is short, say so, give the exact date, and apologize for short notice.

Revise draft bases on co-author input. Re-circulate draft. Expect multiple rounds of drafts, comments and revisions.

The senior author will make the decision when the article is ready to submit to a journal.

Always send the final draft that was submitted externally (conference & journal) to all co-authors

© The Editor(s) (if applicable) and The Author(s) 2022
S. Luby, D. L. Southern, *The Pathway to Publishing: A Guide to Quantitative Writing in the Health Sciences*, https://doi.org/10.1007/978-3-030-98175-4

Appendix 6
High-Level Outline

Use subtitles that match your study.

Limit to ≤1500 words excluding tables, figures, and references.

Introduction
- **Context.**

  – Introduce the subject to provide context for the objective.

- **Knowledge gap.**

  – What don't we know that this manuscript will address?

- **Relevance.**

  – Why is this knowledge important (the "so what?" question).

- **Objective of the manuscript.**

Methods
- **Study site and population.**

  – Outline the setting where the study was carried out, for example, urban versus rural.
  – Mention the study participants, for example, women or children under 5 years of age.

- **Design and sampling.**

  – Describe the study design/approach.
  – Provide key operational definitions.
  – Outline sampling methods.

- **Data collection?**

  – Outline data collection approaches.
  – Outline any special laboratory materials, equipment, or reagents.

© The Editor(s) (if applicable) and The Author(s) 2022
S. Luby, D. L. Southern, *The Pathway to Publishing: A Guide to Quantitative Writing in the Health Sciences*, https://doi.org/10.1007/978-3-030-98175-4

- **Data analysis.**

  – Outline primary approach.

Results
- One bullet point to summarize each table.
- One bullet point to summarize each figure.

Discussion
- **Summary interpretation of overall results.**

  – Link to objectives and rationale.
  – Avoid repeating the results (no statistics).

- **List the primary conclusions that you can logically and defensibly draw from the results.**

  – Outline key arguments that supports this conclusion.
  – If a statistical association represents one of the core conclusions and you believe the association reflects an underlying causal relationship, then outline evidence to support that this association is likely causal. Also outline alternative potential interpretations and evidence that supports them.
  – Focus on internal validity first in the discussion. That is, what conclusions can be drawn soundly about this study population?
  – After discussing internal validity, then discuss external validity. That is, how generalizable are these results and conclusions to other settings? How do these results compare to assessments conducted in other places and times?

- **Limitations.**

  – Focus on the impact that these limitations have on the conclusions we can draw the study.
  – Outline how you interpret the data in light of these limitations.

- **Conclusions**

  – Outline the big picture: How do your results help us understand a broader topic?
  – What implications do your results have for public health or related policies?

- **Recommendations.**

  – What are the key next steps that are practical and applicable to the context?
  – What specific research question should next be pursued?

- **References**

  – Need not be complete but helps clarify the key issues in the introduction and discussion.
  – Permits the author to offer an interpretation based on the literature of key issues and provides the co-authors the opportunity for input on this framing.

- **Tables and figures**

Appendix 7
Example of Quantitative Manuscript HLO

Title: Difficulties in Maintaining Improved Handwashing Behavior, Karachi, Pakistan [17]

Introduction

- Handwashing with soap can reduce diarrhea and respiratory illness *(Refs)*.
- Handwashing promotion that requires repeated household visits is prohibitively expensive on a large scale *(Refs)*.
- In 2003, we conducted a cluster randomized control trial in low-income squatter settlements in Karachi, Pakistan.
- Fieldworkers promoted improved handwashing by providing households with free soap and weekly visits over a 9-month period up to December 2003.
- We conducted a follow-up study 18 months later to determine how long selected households sustained improved handwashing practices.

Methods
Study Setting

- Adjoining multiethnic squatter settlements in central Karachi.
- Fieldwork was conducted by Health-Oriented Preventive Education (HOPE), a local nongovernmental organization.

Study Design

- In the 2003 cluster randomized control trial, 47 clusters of households were selected and randomly assigned 5 intervention groups:

    - 9 clusters received soap and encouragement.
    - 10 clusters received soap, handwashing promotion. and flocculent disinfectant.
    - 9 were controls that received no intervention.

© The Editor(s) (if applicable) and The Author(s) 2022
S. Luby, D. L. Southern, *The Pathway to Publishing: A Guide to Quantitative Writing in the Health Sciences*, https://doi.org/10.1007/978-3-030-98175-4

- In the 2005 follow-up cohort study, fieldworkers, who had not participated in the 2003 study, attempted to revisit households assigned to either of the intervention clusters that included soap and handwashing promotion or to the control group (Figure 1).

Data Collection

- Fieldworkers conducted a re-enrolment survey using a standard questionnaire and performed spot checks of facilities for handwashing.

  - They asked the mother or caregiver of the household:
  - To demonstrate usual handwashing practices.
  - If any children in the household had diarrhea (three or more loose stools within 24 hours) in the preceding week and, if so, for how many days.
  - If mother or caregiver had diarrhea.
  - How much hand soap was purchased in the preceding week.

Data Analysis

- We compared characteristics of re-enrolled households by originally assigned intervention groups with the control group using generalized estimating equation.
- We calculated respondents' longitudinal prevalence of diarrhea.
- To assess the relationship between soap consumption and diarrhea, we used the number of bars of soap purchased during the week divided by the number of persons in the households as the independent variable and the longitudinal prevalence of diarrhea in the subsequent week as a dependent variable in a generalized estimating equation model.
- For all generalized estimating equation models, we used an exchangeable correlation structure applied to neighborhoods to account for clustering derived from spatial proximity.

Results
Descriptive

- A total of 577 households were enrolled: 69% (560) were re-enrolled from the original study's 810 households; 17 were households that split and set up new households in the same study area.
- The 560 re-enrolled households were similar to the 250 households that declined re-enrolment by household size, water supply, reported income, and amount spent on soap and water (Table 1).
- Households that re-enrolled were more likely to have been assigned to the handwashing promotion with soap intervention during the original study and were more likely to own a refrigerator and television (Table 1).

Handwashing Behavior

- At re-enrolment, intervention and control households were just as likely to have soap in the house and reported similar spending on hand soap (Table 2).

- Households originally assigned to handwashing promotion, but with no water treatment, were more likely to have a handwashing station with soap and water (79%) than control households (53%, $P = 0.001$) or households that received both handwashing promotion and water treatment (64% $P = 0.05$).
- During the 63-week follow-up, intervention households purchased a similar quantity of soap and used a similar amount of soap per capita per week compared with control households (Table 2; Figure 2).

Diarrhea Prevalence

- During the first 5 months of follow-up, households from the different intervention groups reported different prevalence of diarrhea. In the subsequent 8 months, the prevalence was similar across the groups (Figure 3).
- The overall longitudinal prevalence of diarrhea was 15–16% lower in the intervention households. After accounting for clustering, neither the longitudinal prevalence among all ages nor any of the age-specific diarrheal prevalence were significantly different between intervention and control households (Table 3).
- There was no association between weekly per capita soap consumption and longitudinal prevalence of household diarrhea in the following week ($P = 0.38$).

Discussion
- These findings illustrate important barriers to improving handwashing behaviors globally. Households that received the handwashing intervention:

  - Acquired the habit of washing hands properly and maintained it for several months.
  - Had a better place to wash hands.
  - Experienced a substantial reduction in diarrhea.

- When soap was no longer provided free, and regular encouragement to wash hands stopped, their behavior reverted to less soap consumption and a disease experience that was no different than households that received no intervention.
- These results are similar to findings from a follow-up of a randomized controlled trial of household water treatment that found high levels of product use during the study period accompanied by a marked reduction in diarrhea but no sustained regular use.

  - Only four evaluations of long-term sustainability of handwashing promotion were identified *(Refs)*.

- In the Karachi study, the lack of a sustained improvement in handwashing behavior suggests that specific methods used for short-term efficacy, for example, free soap, did not produce long-term behavior change.

  - This is consistent with behavior change specialists who note that maintaining a changed behavior is fundamentally different from acquiring a new behavior: Maintenance has different determinants and requires different interventions (Refs).

- In the first 6 months, there was some difference in diarrhea prevalence, but later there was none, suggesting the declining impact of the intervention over time that might have been lessened with occasional refresher visits.
- The amount of soap purchased by households was used as an indirect measure of handwashing, taking into account that soap is used for many household purposes and is sold in different sizes.
  - We hypothesized if handwashing increased, then soap purchases would increase.
  - No difference in amount of soap or an increase in spending on soap suggests no sustained change behavior by this intensive intervention.

Limitations
- Limited power to detect a difference in the longitudinal prevalence of diarrhea between the intervention and control arm.
- Of the originally enrolled households, 29% did not participate in the follow-up evaluation.

Conclusion
- Improved handwashing behavior is not guaranteed to be maintained when the activities promoting that behavior are withdrawn.

Recommendation
- Like other behavior change interventions, maintaining effective handwashing behavior requires focused efforts and research on optimal strategies.

Tables and Figures
Table 1 Comparison of persons re-enrolling versus persons declining re-enrolment
Table 2 Soap use by group among households re-enrolled in August 2005, 20 months after active handwashing promotion and provision of supplies ended
Table 3 Mean longitudinal prevalence of diarrhea by age and intervention group
Figure 1 Study timeline
Figure 2 Bars of soap purchased per person by group and week

Appendix 8
Authorship Scorecard

A Worksheet for Authorship of Scientific Articles.

Author: Robert H. Schmidt

Source: Bulletin of the Ecological Society of America, Vol. 68, No. 1 (Mar., 1987), pp. 8–10 (Included with permission of publisher and author)

Inclusion as an author in a scientific publication is important to many ecologists for reasons of prestige and advancement. Publications are a key factor in deciding on promotion for many ecologists at universities (Jackson and Prato's 1983, Croll 1984). The order of listed authors in a paper is assumed to be an indication of the relative contribution of each of the included authors.

Day (1983, 15–19), Croll (1984), Kennedy (1985), and Jackson (1986) reviewed contemporary difficulties with decision-making in assigning authorship. Dixon et al. (1978) proposed guidelines for determining inclusion and ranking in authorship of a scientific publication. They divided research investigations into five areas, conception (including funding), design, data collection, data analysis, and manuscript preparation, and recommended that authors need to make, at a minimum, a significant contribution in manuscript preparation and in at least one other area. Authorship order was determined by a ranking of the number of areas in which significant contributions were made.

This paper details a method for assisting in (1) deciding who is to be listed as an author on a paper and (2) the ordinal ranking of authors listed on a paper. Of course, the best procedure for dealing with potential problems in assigning authorship is to deal with the issue at the beginning of a study. However, even preassigned roles can have complications especially when personnel in a project change or when responsibilities are transferred. In addition, people often underestimate the inputs required,

© The Editor(s) (if applicable) and The Author(s) 2022
S. Luby, D. L. Southern, *The Pathway to Publishing: A Guide to Quantitative Writing in the Health Sciences*, https://doi.org/10.1007/978-3-030-98175-4

Table A2 Format and example of worksheet for determining the relative contributions of participants in a research project

Investigator	Conception (1.0)	Design (1.0)	Data collection (1.0)	Data analysis (1.0)	Writing (1.0)	Total
Leader A	50	90	0	70	40	250
Leader B	50	10	20	0	30	110
Technician C	0	0	40	30	30	100
Technician D	0	0	40	0	0	40
Column totals	100	100	100	100	100	500

Values listed are percent relative contributions. In this example, a natural cutoff for authorship would be between Technicians C and D. Authorship's rankings should be Leader A, Leader B, and Technician C. The number in parentheses is a multiplier (see text for details)

especially time, for the various contributions making initial agreements, in retrospect, seem unfair. The trend toward multiauthor papers may indicate how research is becoming increasingly interdisciplinary. In these situations, a method for defining authorship roles becomes useful. This simple technique should be a useful decision-making aid, especially for projects with many researchers involved.

A general framework for a decision-making worksheet, with an example, is given in Table A2. For each of the five parts of the research investigation (as defined by Dixon), the relative contribution of each participant is assessed. For each part, total contributions should equal 100%. When all contributions have been assigned, row values are added resulting in a "score" of between 1 and 500. The relative contribution of all participants can then be assessed, and a natural break between subsets of scores on the lower end of the contributions can be used as a cutoff to delineate inclusion as an author. Scores can then be ranked for order of authorship

This technique has a number of assumptions. First, it assumes that each of the five parts of a research investigation are weighted equally. In some situations, this may not be the case. For example, a study may require minimal funding, the infrastructure of a principal investigator's laboratory may be essential to a successful project, or the data set may be collected over several years. This situation is easily dealt with by upgrading the unbalanced part with the multiplier. For example, all of the values in the "data collection" column can be multiplied by 1.2 if data collection is judged to have been 20% more important than the other areas.

Secondly, this technique assumes that all contributions can be judged fairly and accurately. This may not always be the case; indeed, it may be that this technique would only be necessary for papers where it is difficult to assess contributions. Two points are suggested for resolving this. It must first be recognized that each contribution score is usually an estimate and, as such, has some corresponding error associated with it. Therefore, the difference of only a few points between the participant scores is probably not sufficient to rate relative contributions, and other methods must be utilized to determine authorship ranking (perhaps even the flip of a coin). As the second point, a consensus-type survey system, such as the Delphi system

(Schuster et al. 1985), may be useful as an in-house tool for resolving difficult authorship assignment problems although it is recognized that assigning authorship is rarely a democratic process.

How are contributions assessed? One method that could be used is the actual time (hours, days, years) put into each of the five parts of the research investigation. A key problem here is the importance of experience. For example, how would you compare a two-hour contribution to a project's design from a person with 30 years of experience with a 2-hour contribution from a person with little or no experience? Another method admittedly subjective is an assessment of the "importance" (relative to intellection) of contributions in each area. Again, a consensus-type survey can be helpful in arriving at an acceptable and agreeable assessment. The development of some criteria for better assessments or contributions is needed. Time should be minimized, while intellectual contributions should be maximized, yet it is easy to visualize a project in which time is a real measure of effort.

Finally, there is a situation which involves teams of workers involved in one of the five parts. A realistic example would be having many workers assisting in data collection. Although the team's contribution may be large (perhaps 100% of the data collection), the relative contribution of each team member is small. The "points" given to this team may then be assigned to the team coordinator or leader. There is some question whether a "technician" should ever be a co-author, especially if his or her sole responsibility is data collection or data collection and analysis, and the analysis is limited to performing routine operations rather than interpretation (Dixon et al. 1978).

It must be repeated that this system for determining authorship of scientific articles should not replace consultation among authors. However, it should be useful in delineating relative individual contributions when there are many, and it can help project coordinators or senior authors identify personnel who have contributed in a significant way to the study's conclusion. Authorship is a symbol that means taking responsibility for the contents of the paper (Jackson 1986). If the responsibility is there, inclusion as a co-author is appropriate. This worksheet should be helpful in defining this responsibility.

Acknowledgments

For helpful comments on this essay, I thank C. Shugart, W. Howard, J. Aloi, R. Case, T. Tomasi, D. Anderson, R. Johnson, J. Tully, P. Moyle, and T. Salmon.

Literature Cited

Croll, R. P. 1984. The noncontributing author: an issue of credit and responsibility. Perspectives in Biology and Medicine **27**:401–407.

Day, R. A. 1983. How to write and publish a scientific paper. ISI, Philadelphia, Pennsylvania, USA.

Dickson J. D., Conner R. N., Adair K. T. 1978. Guidelines for authorship of scientific articles. Wildlife Society Bulletin **6**:260–261.

Jackson C. I., 1986. Honor in science. Sigma Xi, New Haven, Connecticut, USA.

Jackson C. I., Prados, J. W. 1983. Honor in science. American Scientist **71**:462–464.

Kennedy, D. 1985. On academic authorship. American Council of Learned Societies, Office of Scholarly Communication and Technology, Scholarly Communication Reprint 4:1–5.

Schuster E. G., Frissell S. S., Baker E. E., Lovelass R. S. 1985. The Delphi method: application to elk habitat quality. United States Forest Service Intermountain Research Station Paper. **INT-353**.

Appendix 9
Conference/Scientific Meeting Abstracts

Conference planners often publish a "Call for Abstracts" to identify verbal presentations and posters on relevant subjects that can be featured in that meeting. Before applying, read all the information about the conference carefully. Ensure that the potential audience is the right fit to showcase your particular results. Conference presentations are excellent opportunities to collect feedback on your work. Such feedback can help in the development of your manuscript. You want to choose a conference where the attendees will be interested in your work and so likely to provide thoughtful feedback.

Usually, the conference will give specific guidelines on the length of the abstract and how to submit online. Read all the instructions carefully before developing your abstract. Review examples of accepted abstracts from prior years of the targeted conference. These are generally available online.

You can think of your abstract as a mini-version of your study that includes four sections: background, methods, results, and conclusion. Do not include references. You can use numerals instead of words to save characters and space. But make sure to include your main results, that is, the specific numbers, especially for primary outcome measures.

To develop an abstract, follow these steps in sequence to develop each section:

Step 1: Results
- Present the main findings of the study as specific quantitative results.
- Use your framing document to identify the main results.
- Include raw data including percentages, confidence intervals, odds ratios, p-values, or whatever statistical analysis is appropriate to communicate your results.

Step 2: Conclusion
- Explain what these results mean, that is, what their broader implications are for science or for public health.
- They may support specific public health action or specific next steps in research.
- This is not a summary. Do not repeat the results.

© The Editor(s) (if applicable) and The Author(s) 2022
S. Luby, D. L. Southern, *The Pathway to Publishing: A Guide to Quantitative Writing in the Health Sciences*, https://doi.org/10.1007/978-3-030-98175-4

Step 3: Methods
- Summarize how the study was carried out. Describe the study population and explain the key techniques used to generate the primary results.
- For each result, check that you have included a corresponding method.

Step 4: Background
- Provide key information directly related to your objective and results.
- The last sentence should be a clear statement of your objective. If the word limit is restrictive and there is only space for a single sentence in the background section, then one sentence should be the objective of the study.

Then rearrange the sections to fit into the conference abstract format of background, methods, results, and conclusions. Share with your co-author team and revise until submission.

Review examples of accepted abstracts from prior years of the targeted conference. These are generally available online.

Appendix 10
JANE (Journal/Author Name Estimator)

This information and more and is available on https://jane.biosemantics.org/

Summary

With an exponentially growing number of articles being published every year, scientists can use some help in determining which journal is most appropriate for publishing their results and which other scientists can be called upon to review their work. Jane is a freely available Web-based application that, on the basis of a sample text (e.g., the title and abstract of a manuscript), can suggest journals and experts who have published similar articles [18].

How Does Jane Work?

First, Jane searches for the 50 articles that are most similar to your input. For each of these articles, a similarity score between that article and your input is calculated. The similarity scores of all the articles belonging to a certain journal or author are summed to calculate the confidence score for that journal or author. The results are ranked by confidence score. For more information, you can read.

How Often Is the Data behind Jane Updated?

Currently the data are being updated once every month.

Which Journals Are Included in Jane?

Basically, all journals included in Medline are included in Jane. However, in order to show only active journals, we do not show journals for which no entry was found in Medline in the last year.

Which Authors Are Included in Jane?

All authors that have published one or more articles in the last 10 years that have been included in Medline are included in Jane.

© The Editor(s) (if applicable) and The Author(s) 2022
S. Luby, D. L. Southern, *The Pathway to Publishing: A Guide to Quantitative Writing in the Health Sciences*, https://doi.org/10.1007/978-3-030-98175-4

Which Papers Are Included in Jane?

All records in Medline have been included that (1) contained an abstract, (2) were published in the last 10 years, and (3) did not belong to one of these categories: comment, editorial, news, historical article, congresses, biography, newspaper article, practice guideline, interview, bibliography, legal cases, lectures, consensus development conference, addresses, clinical conference, patient education handout, directory, technical report, festschrift, retraction of publication, retracted publication, duplicate publication, scientific integrity review, published erratum, periodical index, dictionary, and legislation or government publication.

Appendix 11
List of Common Errors

2. General Research and Writing Practices

2.1. Insufficient knowledge of the literature

2.2. Insufficient citations

    2.2.1. Not providing a reference to support an observation

    2.2.2. Plagiarism

2.3. Weak citations

    2.3.1. Citing a secondary source

    2.3.2. Presenting conclusions rather than data from references

    2.3.3. Arguing from authority

2.4. Endnotes not in standard style

    2.4.1. Arguing from authority

    2.4.2. Not proofreading references prior to submission

2.5. Not using standard draft manuscript form

2.6. Repeating information

2.7. Labeling a scientific document as "final"

2.8. Characterizing an observation as "the first"

2.9. Errors in reasoning

    2.9.1. Casual assertion of causality

    2.9.2. Assuming association is causality

    2.9.3. Assuming reported behavior reflects actual behavior

    2.9.4. Confusing imperfect recall with recall bias

    2.9.5. Confusing absence of recognition with absence

    2.9.6. Asserting seasonality with a single year of data

    2.9.7. Drawing conclusions using confirmation bias.

2.10. Constructing a multivariate model using only statistical criteria

© The Editor(s) (if applicable) and The Author(s) 2022
S. Luby, D. L. Southern, *The Pathway to Publishing: A Guide to Quantitative Writing in the Health Sciences*, https://doi.org/10.1007/978-3-030-98175-4

3. Content of Quantitative Papers

3.1. Improper focus or format of title and abstract
3.2. Confusing the role of introduction, methods, results, and discussion
3.3. Not writing the methods section in chronological order
3.4. Not emphasizing steps taken to protect human subjects
3.5. Listing interpretations but not defending one in the discussion
3.6. Not fully explaining limitations
3.7. Writing generic recommendations
3.8. Presenting new data in the discussion
3.9. Reporting the number of enrolled subjects in the methods
3.10. Specifying the contents of a questionnaire
3.11. Naïve theories of change

   3.11.1. Recommending a massive increase in funding
   3.11.2. Ignoring incentives and barriers
   3.11.3. Assuming weak states can implement

3.12. An insufficiently focused introduction
3.13. Failure to clarify key sample size assumptions
3.14. A high-level outline that is not high level
3.15. Specifying software used for routine data analysis
3.16. Presenting rationale in the last sentence of the introduction

4. Mechanics of Writing

4.1. Using nonstandard acronyms
4.2. Using nonstandard spaces
4.3. Improper spelling
4.4. Capitalization problems

   4.4.1. Using all capital letters
   4.4.2. Capitalizing non-proper nouns

4.5. Failure to spell out a numeral <10
4.6. Starting a sentence with a numeral
4.7. Not indenting paragraphs
4.8. Not aligning text to the left
4.9. Problems with parentheses
4.10. Not recognizing when an abbreviation has become a name
4.11. Misplaced commas in large numbers
4.12. Varying fonts within the narrative
4.13. Using bulleted lists rather than sentences
4.14. Uninformative document names

5. Grammatical Structures and Stylistic Strategies

5.1. Using present rather than past tense
5.2. Failure to use definite and indefinite articles
5.3. Excessive use of passive voice
5.4. Improper use of "we"
5.5. Writing from a psychological perspective
5.6. Using excessive subheadings in the discussion
5.7. Misplaced modifiers
5.8. Using nouns with awkward syntax in place of verbs
5.9. Using different terms for the same object or the same idea

6. Achieving Clarity and Conciseness

6.1. Labeling rather than explaining
6.2. Using weak opening phrases for sentences
6.3. Using adjectives and qualifiers
6.4. Overusing studies or authors as sentence subjects
6.5. Using nondescriptive numeric or alphabetical labels
6.6. Using respectively
6.7. Using the word etcetera
6.8. Using a non-English word as an English word
6.9. Describing costs only in local currency
6.10. Using the term "developing country"
6.11. Using the term "socioeconomic status" as a synonym for wealth
6.12. Using technical terms in their nontechnical sense

 6.12.1. Using the term "random" in its nontechnical sense
 6.12.2. Using the term "reliable" in its nontechnical sense
 6.12.3. Using the term "significant" in its nontechnical sense
 6.12.4. Using the term "valid" in its nontechnical sense
 6.12.5. Using the term "incidence" incorrectly
 6.12.6. Using the term "correlated" incorrectly

6.13. Using the term "documented"
6.14. Framing an argument in terms of need
6.15. Using the term "illiterate" as a synonym for "no formal education"
6.16. Using "challenging" as a synonym for "difficult"
6.17. Describing a laboratory test result as positive
6.18. Using increase or decrease in the absence of a time trend
6.19. Describing a test as a gold standard

7. Recording Scientific Data

7.1. Using statistics in place of the study question to frame results

 7.1.1. Framing narrative results around p-values

7.2. Not presenting the core data

7.3. Using too many decimal places

7.4. Using too few decimal places

7.5. Using incomplete headings for tables and figures

7.6. Imbalance between table and narrative presentation of the results

> 7.6.1. Too little narratives explaining the table
>
> 7.6.2. Too much narrative explaining the table
>
> 7.6.3. Presenting results in narrative that would be clearer in a table

7.7. Pointing too explicitly to tables and figures

7.8. Using inappropriate figures

7.9. Generic tables that lack a clear message

7.10. Table layout that impairs comparisons

7.11. Using less informative denominators in a table

7.12. Comparing to a varying baseline

7.13. P-value in a baseline table of a randomized controlled trial

7.14. Using nonstandard footnote symbols in tables

7.15. Using the wrong symbol to designate degree

7.16. Numbering figures or tables out of sequence

7.17. Maps with irrelevant details

8. Approaching Publication.

8.1. Failure to respond to reviewers' comments

8.2. Incomplete response to external reviews

> 8.2.1. Not including text of the manuscript changes in response to external reviewers

8.3. Invalid authorship line

8.4. Retaining comments in subsequent drafts

8.5. Choosing an inappropriate journal

8.6. Not following a specific journal's details of style

8.7. Not using an appropriate reporting guideline

8.8. Exceeding the journal word limit

8.9. Asking your senior author to recommend reviewers

8.10. Responding to journal reviewers using the first person singular

8.11. Missing acknowledgment section

8.12. Reusing an email thread when circulating a revised manuscript

8.13. Requesting an unprofessionally short turnaround time

8.14. Sending black forms for co-authors to complete

8.15. Not providing co-authors a copy of the submitted manuscript

8.16. Not keeping co-authors informed of journal discussions

8.17. Emailing draft manuscripts with figures that are not compressed

8.18. Not including readability statistics

9. Slide presentations

9.1. Bullets on the wall
9.2. Using sentences for bullet points
9.3. Too much space between bullets
9.4. Using bullets without hanging indents
9.5. Chart junk
9.6. Using three-dimensional chart features as decorations.
9.7. Using a pie chart.
9.8. Using vertical bars when horizontal bars would communicate better.
9.9. Copying a manuscript figure instead of developing a custom figure
9.10. Photos with an unnatural aspect ratio
9.11. Too many photographs on a single slide
9.12. Fieldworkers as the dominant subject of photographs
9.13. Including a final "Thank You" slide
9.14. Failure to separate ideas in a multilined title

References

1. Hill AB. The environment and disease: association or causation? Proc R Soc Med. 1965;58:295–300.
2. Bernard HR, Killworth P, Kronenfeld D, Sailer L. The problem of informant accuracy: the validity of retrospective data. Annu Rev Anthropol. 1984;13:495–517.
3. Manun'Ebo M, Cousens S, Haggerty P, Kalengaie M, Ashworth A, Kirkwood B. Measuring hygiene practices: a comparison of questionnaires with direct observations in rural Zaire. Tropical Med Int Health. 1997;2:1015–21.
4. Curtis V, Cousens S, Mertens T, Traore E, Kanki B, Diallo I. Structured observations of hygiene behaviours in Burkina Faso: validity, variability, and utility. Bull World Health Organ. 1993;71:23–32.
5. Halder AK, Tronchet C, Akhter S, Bhuiya A, Johnston R, Luby SP. Observed hand cleanliness and other measures of handwashing behavior in rural Bangladesh. BMC Public Health. 2010;10:545.
6. Pedersen DM, Keithly S, Brady K. Effects of an observer on conformity to handwashing norm. Percept Mot Skills. 1986;62:169–70.
7. Munger K, Harris SJ. Effects of an observer on handwashing in a public restroom. Percept Mot Skills. 1989;69:733–4.
8. Drankiewicz D, Dundes L. Handwashing among female college students. Am J Infect Control. 2003;31:67–71.
9. Ram PK, Halder AK, Granger SP, et al. Is structured observation a valid technique to measure handwashing behavior? Use of acceleration sensors embedded in soap to assess reactivity to structured observation. Am J Trop Med Hyg. 2010;83:1070–6.
10. Nickerson RS. Confirmation bias: a ubiquitous phenomenon in many guises. Rev Gen Psychol. 1998;2:175.
11. VanderWeele T, Staudt N. Causal diagrams for empirical legal research: a methodology for identifying causation, avoiding bias and interpreting results. Law Probab Risk. 2011;10:329–54.
12. Robins JM. Data, design, and background knowledge in etiologic inference. Epidemiology. 2001;12:313–20.
13. Greenland S, Pearl J, Robins JM. Causal diagrams for epidemiologic research. Epidemiology. 1999;10:37–48.

© The Editor(s) (if applicable) and The Author(s) 2022
S. Luby, D. L. Southern, *The Pathway to Publishing: A Guide to Quantitative Writing in the Health Sciences*, https://doi.org/10.1007/978-3-030-98175-4

14. Carpenter DP. The forging of bureaucratic autonomy: reputations, networks, and policy innovation in executive agencies, 1862–1928. Princeton: Princeton University Press; 2001.
15. Chavalarias D, Wallach JD, Li AH, Ioannidis JP. Evolution of reporting P values in the biomedical literature, 1990-2015. JAMA. 2016;315:1141–8.
16. Ehrenberg ASC. Rudiments of numeracy. J. R Stat Soc Ser A (Gen). 1977;140:277–97.
17. Luby SP, Agboatwalla M, Bowen A, Kenah E, Sharker Y, Hoekstra RM. Difficulties in maintaining improved handwashing behavior, Karachi, Pakistan. Am J Trop Med Hyg. 2009;81:140–5.
18. Schuemie M, Kors J. Jane: suggesting journals, finding experts. Bioinformatics. 2008;24:727–8.

Printed in the United States
by Baker & Taylor Publisher Services